Oklahoma Notes

Clinical Sciences Review for Medical Licensure
Developed at
The University of Oklahoma College of Medicine

Ronald S. Krug, *Series Editor*

Suitable Reviews for:
United States Medical Licensing Examination (USMLE), Step 2
Federation Licensing Examination (FLEX)

Oklahoma Notes

Obstetrics and Gynecology

Pamela S. Miles
William F. Rayburn
J. Christopher Carey

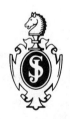

Springer-Verlag
New York Berlin Heidelberg London Paris
Tokyo Hong Kong Barcelona Budapest

Pamela S. Miles, M.D.
Department of Obstetrics
    and Gynecology
Health Sciences Center
The University of Oklahoma
Oklahoma City, OK 73190
USA

William F. Rayburn, M.D.
Department of Obstetrics
    and Gynecology
Health Sciences Center
The University of Oklahoma
Oklahoma City, OK 73190
USA

J. Christopher Carey, M.D.
Department of Obstetrics
    and Gynecology
Health Sciences Center
The University of Oklahoma
Oklahoma City, OK 73190
USA

Library of Congress Cataloging-in-Publication Data
    available upon request.

Printed on acid-free paper.

Production managed by Jim Harbison; manufacturing supervised by Jacqui Ashri.
Camera-ready copy prepared by the authors.
Printed and bound by Edwards Brothers, Inc., Ann Arbor, MI.
Printed in the United States of America.

9 8 7 6 5 4 3 2

ISBN 0-387-94184-3 Springer-Verlag New York Berlin Heidelberg
ISBN 3-540-94184-3 Springer-Verlag Berlin Heidelberg New York

Preface to the
Oklahoma Notes

In 1973 the University of Oklahoma College of Medicine instituted a requirement for passage of the Part 1 National Boards for promotion to the third year. To assist students in preparation for this examination a two-week review of the basic sciences was added to the Curriculum in 1975. Ten review texts were written by the faculty. In 1987 these basic science review texts were published as the *Oklahoma Notes* ("Okie Notes") and made available to all students of medicine who were preparing for comprehensive examinations. Over a quarter of a million of these texts have been sold nationally. Their clear, concise outline format has been found to be extremely useful by students preparing themselves for nationally standardized examinations.

Over the past few years numerous inquiries have been made regarding the availability of a Clinical Years series of "Okie Notes." Because of the obvious utility of the basic sciences books, faculty associated with the University of Oklahoma College of Medicine have developed texts in five specialty areas: Medicine, Neurology, Pediatrics, Psychiatry, and Surgery. Each of these texts follows the same condensed outline format as the basic science texts. The faculty who have prepared these texts are clinical educators and therefore the material incorporated in these texts has been validated in the classroom.

Each author has endeavored to distill the "need to know" material from their field of expertise. While preparing these texts, the target audience has always been the clinical years student who is preparing for Step 2 examinations.

A great deal of effort has gone into these texts. I hope they are helpful to you in studying for your licensure examinations.

Ronald S. Krug, Ph.D.
Series Editor

Preface

This book is intended to be a study guide in preparing for student level examinations in obstetrics and gynecology. We used the medical student educational objectives provided by the Association of Professors in Gynecology and Obstetrics to serve as a guideline for the information we included in the book. With these as a guide, we hope to provide uniform information that all medical students are expected to know at the completion of their training. We hope this serves as a foundation of information in obstetrics and gynecology that you may always find useful in whatever specialty you pursue.

Pamela S. Miles, M.D.
William F. Rayburn, M.D.
J. Christopher Carey, M.D.

Acknowledgments

We would like to express our gratitude to all of our colleagues in the Obstetrics and Gynecology Department at The University of Oklahoma Health Sciences Center who contributed their knowledge to the writing of this book. Special gratitude goes to Mary Long who has helped us with her wonderful secretarial skills from the very beginning. Additional thanks to Leslie Hudson and Lisa Harris for helping us finish the project. Thanks also to the other secretaries in the Department who contributed work from their sections. The original artwork in the book was done by Lora Carter, and we thank her for lending her talented skills.

Contents

INITIAL PATIENT INTERACTION

COMMUNICATION SKILLS

Goal is to establish a good working relationship with the patient and all members of the health care team

I. Patient

A. Initial introduction to the patient should use the patient's surname to show your respect. After a lengthy relationship has been established, it may be appropriate to use their first name

B. When taking the history, allow the patient to verbalize initially without directed questioning. Maintain eye contact and limit writing

C. During examinations, patient modesty should be considered when draping. "Talking before touching" is a good rule to use. Be conscious of phrases and terminology used during exam.

D. Always maintain patient confidentiality. The patient should give permission for others to share in their medical information and decisions. They may choose to bring family in for support. Confidentiality includes minors in the doctor-patient relationship.

II. Health Care Team

A. Maintain relationship of respect for colleagues and support services personnel. For example, using correct titles, answering pages and calls in a timely fashion

B. Services needed should be delegated to the appropriate provider

C. Keep lines of communication open between providers for the benefit of the patient

III. Physician Limitations

A. The physician should be aware of the limits of his abilities

B. Be aware of the perception and management ideas that may be influenced by one's own sexuality

C. Behavior patterns of seductive patients

HISTORY

I.   Chief Complaint - the reasons for the patient's visit expressed in their own words

II.   Present Illness - a more detailed explanation of the current problem to include physician inquiries

III. Menstrual History

    A.   Age of menarche
    B.   Last menstrual period
    C.   Cycle interval
    D.   Duration and amount of flow
    E.   Associated cyclic symptoms

IV.   Gynecologic History

    A.   Prior diagnosis of gynecologic disease
    B.   Sexually transmitted disease
    C.   Gynecologic surgery
    D.   Pelvic pain
    E.   Vulvar or vaginal lesions
    F.   Pap smear history
    G.   Infertility

V.   Obstetric History

    A.   Gravida - number of total pregnancies

    B.   Para - number of term deliveries; followed by
        1.   Number of preterm
        2.   Number of abortions/miscarriages
        3.   Then number of living children
        4.   Example: G4P2022

    C.   Outcome of each delivery, mode of delivery and any complications should be recorded

VI.   Contraceptive History

    A.   Current contraceptive method

    B.   Length of use and any problems with current method should be recorded

    C.   All prior contraceptive methods and any complications with these should be discussed

VII. **Sexual History**

    A.   Age of first intercourse

    B.   Number of partners

    C.   Known exposure to STD's

    D.   Current problems in sexual function and any history of sexual abuse

VIII. **General Medical History**

    A.   Medications

    B.   Allergies

    C.   Other medical diagnosis

    D.   Past non-gynecologic surgeries

    E.   Social history

    F.   Family history (especially gynecologic or breast disease, genetics

    G.   General review of systems

ROUTINE EXAMINATION

I.   **Goal** is to establish rapport with the patient.

II.   **Breast**

    A.   Inspection - alterations in the appearance of the breast such as changes in shape, contour, symmetry, coloration, skin retractions, or edema

    B.   Palpation - examine the axilla and the entire area of the breast tissue with the flat part of the fingers. A circular pattern moving inwards towards the areola is traditionally used. Any masses felt should be documented in location, consistency, size, shape, and mobility. Gentle pressure on the areola is used to check for any discharge.

III.   **Abdomen**

    A.   Inspection for
        1.   Shape
        2.   Scars
        3.   Striae
        4.   Hair pattern

    B.   Auscultation - for character of bowel sounds

    C.   Palpation for
        1.   Tenderness
        2.   Masses
        3.   Consistency

    D.   Percussion to
        1.   Outline solid organs
        2.   Fluid waves

IV.   **Pelvis** - The history should aid in selection of the appropriate speculum based on patient parity and sexual history. Determination of any tests in addition to the pap should be agreed upon. The patient should be appropriately draped. Head of table elevated about 30" and the patient assisted into the lithotomy position with appropriate lighting available

    A.   Inspection - external genitalia to include
        1.   Mons pubis
        2.   Labia majora
        3.   Labia minora
        4.   Perineum and perianal area
        5.   Urethral meatus
        6.   Clitoris
        7.   Skein's gland and Bartholin's gland areas will be visible for inspection as palpation is begun

8. The vaginal walls and the cervix likewise will be visible after insertion of the speculum

9. A Valsalva maneuver will allow a cystocele or rectocele to be seen

B. Palpation includes
   1. Bartholin's gland
   2. Urethra
   3. Any areas of abnormal appearance

C. Speculum - appropriate speculum placed and cervix and upper vagina visualized. Necessary sampling done
   1. Pap
   2. Cultures
   3. Discharge for wet prep
   4. Any endocervical, cervical or endometrial biopsies needed are taken

D. Bimanual

   1. Abdominal and vaginal hands are used to outline the pelvic structure

   2. The flexion, size, consistency, and tenderness of the uterus are noted - the normal size is 4x6 cm and weights 70 gm.

   3. The adnexal regions are palpated for ovarian size, tenderness, presence of masses, and mobility - normal ovaries during reproductive years are approximately 2.5 cm. Postmenopausal ovaries are usually not palpable

   4. The rectovaginal exam will evaluate the posterior aspect of the uterus, confirm any adnexal masses and allow sampling of stool for occult blood. The bimanual exam also aids evaluate of pelvic support structures

ASSESSMENT AND MANAGEMENT PLAN

I.   Goal - Identify problems and outline an organized plan of evaluation and management

II.   Create a problem list based on history and examination

III.   For each problem, create a list of differential diagnoses

IV.   Select appropriate laboratory testing and diagnostic studies to help confirm or rule out possible diagnosis

V.   Develop a plan of management for each problem

VI.   Incorporate patient education into the management plan; include preventive care

VII.   Set long-term goals for follow-up management

VIII.   Be considerate of patient economic and cultural concerns in the care plan

PREVENTIVE CARE

I. Laboratory Screening

A. Pap smears

1. Recommends beginning at age 18 or sexual activity, whichever happens first

2. After 3 consecutive normal annual exams and Paps, the interval may be increased at the physician's and patient's discretion

B. Mammograms
1. With a negative family history, begin screening mammograms at age 40
2. Should be performed every 1-2 years until age 50.
3. After age 50, they should be done annually.
4. Breast exams should be performed annually at all ages

C. Blood pressure
1. Should be performed as part of an annual exam at all ages

D. Blood lipid profiles
1. Every 5 years

E. Fecal occult blood test
1. Annual beginning at age 40

II. Historical Screening

A. Dietary/nutritional assessment
1. Ideal body weight should be established
2. Balanced diet discussed and plans coordinated with a dietician/nutritionist as needed

B. Exercise program

C. Substance use/abuse
1. Includes use of tobacco, alcohol, and drugs (both prescription and non-prescription)

D. Immunizations
1. Initial history should reveal all routine immunizations were received
2. Women in reproductive years should especially be evaluated for rubella immunity
3. Influenza vaccine should be offered beginning at age 55
4. Tetanus booster is every 10 years.
5. Hepatitis B vaccine should be offered to high risk groups

E.   Stress management
1.   Family and personal relationships should be evaluated
2.   Job satisfaction and work relationships should be discussed

F.   Sexual function
1.   Methods of preventing sexual diseases and pregnancy should be reviewed at each visit

NORMAL OBSTETRICS

PHYSIOLOGIC CHANGES OF PREGNANCY

Three underlying FACTORS which explain physiologic changes seen during pregnancy include:

1. Placental hormones: estrogen (E), progesterone (P), human placental lactogen (HPL)
2. Expanding intravascular volume (V)
3. Compression from the enlarging gravid uterus (C)

SYSTEM/ORGAN	ANATOMIC/PHYSIOLOGIC CHANGE (FACTOR)	SIGNS AND SYMPTOMS LABORATORY CHANGES	PATHOPHYSIOLOGIC CHANGES
Reproduction			
Placenta	Increased size	↑ alkaline phosphatase	abruption
Vulva/Vagina	Congestion (V,C)	Pressure, fullness, swelling	Varicosities
Cervix	Congestion (V,C.) Eversion (E)	Cyanosis, pelvic fullness, vaginal discharge	Pap smear-inflammatory changes,dysplasia
Uterus	Enlargement (P)	Pelvic and ligament pain, weight gain	Uterine anomalies, leiomyoma enlargement
Ovaries	Regression (E,P)	↓ FSH, LH	Luteal cyst, theca lutein cysts
Breast	Stimulation of alveoli (H, HPL) Congestion (V)	Tenderness, enlargement, nipple enlargement	Pain from engorgement, impaired diagnosis

SYSTEM/ORGAN	ANATOMIC/PHYSIOLOGIC CHANGE (FACTOR)	SIGNS AND SYMPTOMS LABORATORY CHANGES	PATHOPHYSIOLOGIC CHANGES
Gastrointestinal			
Salivary glands	Congestion (V)	Ptyalism	Nausea
Gastric	Hyperacidity (E,P) Delayed emptying (C,P)	Dyspepsia, nausea	Hiatal hernia, reflex esophagitis
Hepatic	↑ Protein synthesis (E,P)	↑ albumin, carrier proteins, fibrinogen	Fatty liver, toxemic liver disease
Gall bladder	Delayed emptying (P)	No change in transaminases	Cholestasis, cholecystitis-lithiasis
Intestinal	Delayed emptying (P)	Constipation	Abdominal pain
Rectal/Anal	Venous congestion (V,C)	Hemorrhoids	Thrombosed hemorrhoids
Cardiovascular			
Heart	Cardiomegaly (V), increased cardiac output, heart rate, stroke volume (V)	Enlarged heart on CXR, holosystolic murmur (gr II/VI), palpitation	Cardiomyopathy
Arteries	Smooth muscle relaxation (P), decreased vascular resistance (P)	Hypotension	Pregnancy-induced hypertension
Veins	Congestion (V,C); compression of vena cava (C)	Varicosities, dependent edema, supine hypotension	Thrombophlebitis, edema of hands and face

SYSTEM/ORGAN	ANATOMIC/PHYSIOLOGIC CHANGE (FACTOR)	SIGNS AND SYMPTOMS LABORATORY CHANGES	PATHOPHYSIOLOGIC CHANGES
Respiratory			
Nasal passages	Congestion (V)	Difficulty breathing, nosebleeds, snoring	Upper respiratory infection, nosebleeds
Trachea/Bronchi	Congestion (V)	Dyspnea in cold weather	Asthma
Lungs	Elevation of diaphragm (C)	Dyspnea in late gestation	Pneumonia
Nervous			
Central	Unaffected	Headache (E, V)	Seizures, migraine headaches
Peripheral	Compression (V,C)	Paresthesia (femoral n., ulna n)	Carpal tunnel, sciatica, leg pain
Urinary			
Kidneys	Increased GFR, RBF (V), compression of renal vessels	Proteinuria, glycosuria, urinary frequency	Pyelonephritis
Ureters	Urine stasis (P,C)	Dilation on USN, IVP; ascending bacteruria	Urinary tract infection
Bladder	Urinary frequency (C), Urinary stasis (P)	Bacteruria	Urinary tract infection

SYSTEM/ORGAN	ANATOMIC/PHYSIOLOGIC CHANGE (FACTOR)	SIGNS AND SYMPTOMS LABORATORY CHANGES	PATHOPHYSIOLOGIC CHANGES
Endocrine			
Pituitary			
Anterior	Congestion (V); hypertrophy (P,E)	↓ FSH, LH; ↑ PRL; no ↑ TSH, ACTH	Blurred vision, headaches
Posterior	Oxytocin release	Uterine contractions from nipple stimulation	Shehan's syndrome (excess hemorrhage at delivery)
Thyroid	Thyromegaly (E, ↑ TBG)	↑ TBG, total T4; no change in free T4	Hyperthyroid
Pancreas	Islet cell hyperplasia (H,E,P)	Fasting hypoglycemia	Glucose intolerance
Adrenal	↑ sensitivity to angiotensin (E,P) ↑ aldosterone (P)	↑ CBG, ↑ total cortisol; sodium retention, edema	Hypertension
Musculoskeletal			
Spine	Postural change (C); forward center of gravity (C)	Difficulty in exercising, backache	Severe backache
Extremities	Pressure on legs (C, V)	Swelling, decreased mobility	Excess swelling
Skin	Hormonal effects (P, E), stretching (C)	Spider angioma; Striae, pruritus	Chloasma, umbilical hernia, gestational pruritus

ANTEPARTUM CARE

I.   Diagnosis of Pregnancy

    A.   Presumptive evidence of pregnancy
        1.   Cessation of menses
        2.   Breast changes
        3.   Congestion of the vagina
        4.   Skin changes
        5.   Nausea
        6.   Bladder irritability
        7.   Fatigue
        8.   Perception of fetal movement

    B.   Probable evidence of pregnancy
        1.   Enlargement of the abdomen
        2.   Uterine changes (size, shape, consistency)
        3.   Cervical changes
        4.   Palpationof the fetus
        5.   Braxton Hicks contractions
        6.   Endocrine tests

    C.   Positive evidence of pregnancy
        1.   Demonstration of the fetal heart
        2.   Examiner appreciation of fetal movement
        3.   Visualization of the fetus

II.   Gestational Age Determination

    A.   Last menstrual period
        1.   Add 280 days to first of LMP to get EDC
        2.   If known with certainty, it is the most reliable clinical estimator of gestational age
        3.   Uncertain in 14-58% (average 40%) of all pregnancies
        4.   Nagle's rule - LMP minus 3 months plus 1 weeks to get EDC

    B   Trimesters
        1.   First trimester up to 12-14 weeks
        2.   Second trimester 14-28 weeks
        3.   Third trimester 29-40 weeks.

C.   Initial positive pregnancy test
       1.   Measuring human chorionic gonadotropin
       2.   Types of tests:

Method	Detectable (+) result (postconception)	Test sensitivity mIU/ml

Immunoassay
  Hemagglutination inhibitor*
  Enzyme immunoassay
	
	3-4 weeks
	2 weeks
		
		750-3500
		25 (serum) -50 (urine)

Radioreceptor assay (RRA)	2-3 weeks	100-200

Radioimmunossay (RIA)
  Rapid, qualitative
  24-48 hr, quantitative
	
	2 weeks
	1 week
		
		20-40
		2-4

C.   Initial uterine examination
       1.   terine size may be larger than dates in the presence of a full bladder, trophoblastic disease, uterine fibroids, and twins

D.   Fetal heart rate auscultation
       1.   Amplified (Doppler) auscultation: by 12 weeks
       2.   Unamplified heart sounds: by 20 weeks

E.   Initial perception of fetal movements
       1.   Primigravid: by 19-20 weeks
       2.   Multigravid: by 17-18 weeks.

F.   Uterine fundal height examinations
       1.   Excellent correlation between fundal height measurement (in centimeters) from the upper symphysis to fundus and gestational age (in weeks) between 18-30 weeks; fundus at the level of the umbilicus at 20 weeks

G.   Ultrasonography
       1.   To confirm pregnancy dating if menstrual dates are in question, obstetrical intervention or elective delivery is likely to be required later, or uterine size-date discrepancy exists.
       2.   Early anatomic landmarks include measurements of the gestational sac between 6-10 weeks and crown-rump length between 7-12 weeks.
       3.   The crown-rump length (CRL) in centimeters plus 6.5 approximates the estimated gestational age
       4.   Beyond the 12th week, the most accurate assessment is obtained by averaging different body part measurements (biometry)
            a.   Biparietal diameter (BPD), cerebellum diameter, occipitofrontal diameterabdominal circumference, and femur length

III.   Routine Visits

A.   Evaluations include:
1. Patient interview
2. Weight
3. Blood pressure
4. Urine dipstick for protein and glucose
5. Fetal heart tones
6. Measurements
7. Palpations - Leopolds

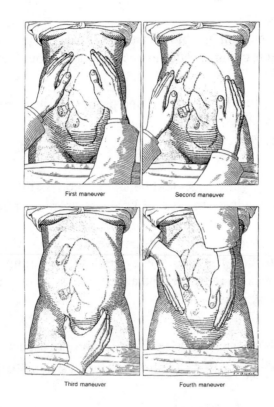

First maneuver   Second maneuver

Third maneuver   Fourth maneuver

From <u>Williams</u> <u>Obstetrics</u>, 19th ed., Appleton & Lange, 1993

B.   Visit interval
1. Every four weeks up to approximately 30 weeks
2. Every two weeks between 30-36 weeks
3. Weekly after 36 weeks

IV. Recommendations to Patients

A. Symptoms during pregnancy

1. Nausea
   a. A usually normal and favorable sign of a health pregnancy
   b. Simple nausea is often treated expectantly with reassurance and diet manipulation
   c. Prenatal vitamins, antihistamines, or both may be helpful
   d. Persistent vomiting requires stronger antiemetic therapy to avoid maternal dehydration, weight loss, and electrolyte imbalance

2. Breast tenderness
   a. Another frequent symptom that occurs early in pregnancy
   b. Lactation is common later in gestation and should not be alarming

3. Fatigue
   a. Daily rest with frequent naps and proper nutrition are necessary
   b. A daily routine of exercise, such as walking, swimming, or bicycling, is recommended

4. Weight gain
   a. Average weight gain should be 30 lbs.; no less than 20 pounds
   b. Some may gain as much as 40 pounds or more if begun under ideal body weight
   c. A gain of more than 2 pounds per week suggests fluid retention
   d. Good nutrition does not necessarily mean eating excessively. Several small snacks or three well-balanced meals per day and a late night snack are recommended

5. Pain
   a. Back, pelvic, and even leg pain are common, especially in late pregnancy
   b. Lying on the side or a change in posture will usually give relief

6. Edema
   a. May occur in the feet and legs
   b. Support pantyhose may be worn while working and standing
   c. Important to note whether any rings become tight and difficult to remove or if there is any swelling of the face, particularly in the morning

7. Urinary frequency
   a. One of the earliest signs of pregnancy
   b. Should expect to awaken several times to empty bladder
   c. Suspect an infection if any burning or pain in the bladder

8. Nasal congestion
   a. Decongestants and antihistamines are used frequently, without added risk
   b. Bleeding of the nose may occasionally accompany

9. Heartburn
   a. Avoid smoking, drinking caffeinated beverages, and lying down after a meal
   b. The entire head of the bed (not just her head) should be elevated

10. Constipation
    a. Due in part to the iron content of vitamin pills, absorption of more fluids into the bloodstream, and compression of the bowel by the enlarging uterus
    b. Helped by increasing fluid intake, eating high fiber foods, and ingesting cellulose powders

11. Hemorrhoids
    a. Rarely require surgery
    b. Usually subside after delivery
    c. Preparation H, Anusol, or Tucks may be used

12. Clothes
    a. Loose fitting and comfortable
    b. Shoes should be comfortable, allowing for modest swelling and provides stability

13 Vaginal discharge
   a. Normal to expect during early and late pregnancy
   b. Evaluate if an increase in discharge, change in color or odor, staining or crusting on undergarments, or itching on the lips of the vagina

B. Precautions to take

1. Diet
   a. Recommend fresh fruit, fresh vegetables, lean meats (chicken, fish), and low-fat dairy products
   b. Intolerance to milk is common during pregnancy. May substitute cheese or yogurt or add chocolate to the milk
   c. Vitamin supplements are not essential during pregnancy as long as nutrition is adequate
   d. Fluoride content in most water supplies is usually sufficient
   e. Iron supplementation is necessary
   f. Caffeinated beverages, such as colas, tea, and coffee, may be ingested in moderation during pregnancy

2. Drugs
   a. Any drugs taken before pregnancy, during early pregnancy, or throughout pregnancy should be sought
   b. Those prescribed for a medical illness may still be necessary and should be taken

3   Smoking and alcohol

    a.   Infants born to mothers who smoke have gained an average of 200 gm (5 oz) less than babies born to nonsmokers

    b.   If the patient is unable to quit, we strongly recommend that she smoke less than 1/2 pack per day and that the cigarettes contain the least nicotine content

    c.   No absolute safe level of ingestion of alcohol during pregnancy

    d.   Signs of the fetal alcohol syndrome require excessive consumption (five or more hard drinks per day) for prolonged periods of time

4.   Sex

    a.   Becomes more difficult, more tiring, and sometimes uncomfortable

    b.   No reason to usually discontinue sexual activity, because it is generally believed not to pose any risk to the fetus or result in an increased risk of premature labor

    c.   If any signs of an abnormal vaginal discharge, any vaginal bleeding, or any leakage of fluid, abstaining from sexual activity would be appropriate

5.   Lightheaded

    a.   Particularly late in pregnancy

    b.   When changing positions from lying down to standing, sitting to standing, and getting out of the bathtub

    c.   Often from hypoglycemia, hypotension, or overexertion

6.   Dental care

    a.   Encouraged during pregnancy

    b.   Much manipulation or surgery should be discussed beforehand

7.   Exercise

    a.   Exercises for childbirth will be taught during childbirth classes.

    b.   Daily walks are to be encouraged.

    c.   Swimming and bicycling are also excellent

    d.   Uterine contractility is not thought to increase with moderate exercise, and any fetal heart rate changes are uncommon and thought to be transient

    e.   Should there be a medical complication, the patient should abstain from vigorous exercise

    f.   The patient should program a time in which she lies on her side (preferably left side) for a minimum of 1 hour each day

8.   Recurrence risks

Complication	Recurrence risk	
Hydatidiform mole	1.3 2.9%	
Recurrent miscarriage	20 - 30%	
Ectopic pregnancy	50%	involuntary infertility
	35 - 40%	successful pregnancy
	10 - 15%	recurrent ectopic
Mild preeclampsia	2.0%	severe preeclampsia
	29.0%	mild preeclampsia
Severe preeclampsia	7.5%	severe preeclampsia
	30.0%	mild preeclampsia
Placental abruption	15%	
Preterm labor x 1	15%	
x 2	30%	
Gestational diabetes	27 -75%	

9.   Advanced maternal age

a.   6% of births in the United States are among women age 35 or older

b.   Appears to be a greater risk of spontaneous abortion, and the stillbirth rate seems to double by the late 30's and increases to three - to four-fold by the mid 40's

c.   Chromosomal abnormalities, especially trisomies 13, 18, and 21, and sex chromosomal aneuploidies increase logarithmically with maternal age starting in the 30's

d.   Bleeding from a placenta previa or abruptio placenta is also thought to be more common

e.   Hypertension, preeclampsia, and diabetes are not only more common but seem to carry an even greater risk

f.   More problems with abnormal labor patterns and a higher incidence of cesarean section

10.   Amniocentesis

a.   For genetic reasons or before delivery to determine fetal lung maturity

b.   Sonogram is usually performed beforehand to localize the placenta and vital fetal parts

c.   Risk to the fetus is very low (one in 250-500 cases shown signs of infection, bleeding, or fetal death)

11.   Travel

a.   Discourage long trips within the last month

b.   A vaginal examination before leaving to determine the dilation of the cervix and provide the name of a competent obstetrician in the community to be visited

c.   If travel is by automobile, one stop is recommended at least every 2 hours to walk and void

d.   It is safe to fly during pregnancy

12. Vaginal bleeding
   a. Should be reported
   b. Common for spotting to occur after sex or a pelvic examination

13. Uterine contractions
   a. Common within three months before the "due date" but should be sought
   b. Irregular contractions occurring less frequently than every 8 minutes are particularly common probably represent Braxton-Hicks contractions.
   c. The physician should be notified if these persist and are as frequent as every 5 minutes despite rest

14. X-rays
   a. Any risk to the fetus is highly unlikely, and there is no indication for a therapeutic abortion
   b. Should these be necessary (such as a chest x-ray or abdominal film), shield the uterus
   c. Usually result in doses much less than 5 rads
   d. A dose of about 10 rads is the lowest associated with structural embryonic or fetal defects

15. Fevers
   a. May be a flu-like illness or represent a more serious infection such as pyelonephritis or pneumonia
   b. Actual harm to the fetus from high fevers cannot be clearly determined

16. Venereal infections
   a. Any prior gonorrhea, syphilis, herpes, or chlamydia should be reported
   b. Further tests may be necessary

17. Headaches
   a. Common during pregnancy
   b. Persistent headaches associated with high blood pressure are often accompanied with dimming and blurring of vision and spots being seen

18. Abdominal pain
   a. Common to have occasional abdominal cramps that are related to Braxton-Hicks uterine contractions
   b. Should remain at rest if the cramping persists
   c. May be associated with a placental separation from the uterine wall (abruptio placenta) or premature labor

19. Fluid from the vagina
   a. Either a loss of urine, cervical discharge, or rupture of the amniotic membranes
   b. Usually occurs within the last 2 months of pregnancy

20 Decrease in fetal movement
   a. May merely represent more coordinated movements ("rollover") rather than simple kicks

b. Documented fetal inactivity suggests distress and requires further biophysical evaluation

c. A patient is asked to keep a daily record of the fetus' activity during at least one convenient hour of monitoring while lying on her side

C. Preparing for childbirth and infant care

1. Childbirth classes

   a. Strongly encouraged to attend

   b. Discuss any concerns

   c. Discuss what to expect during labor and delivery and what may be used for pain relief

   d. If prior cesarean section, every effort can be made to attempt a vaginal birth experience if the patient and her spouse desire

2 Options available during labor and delivery

   a. Electronic fetal heart monitoring, vaginal prep, sibling visitation, 24-hour rooming-in, early hospital discharge, and visiting nurse home visits

   b. Hospitals usually provide "birthing rooms" in which the mother can both labor and deliver

   c. A "birthing room" may decrease the admission-to-delivery interval, decrease the analgesia requirement, allow more freedom of movement, increase rooming-in time, and decrease hospital costs

3. Circumcision

   a. Encourage that you seek her thoughts on circumcision before labor

   b. Although the complication rate is very low, a circumcision is cosmetic and not absolutely medically necessary

4. Baby's doctor

   a. Encourage a pediatrician of family physician to be chosen beforehand

   b. The baby's first visit should be scheduled usually for the second week after delivery

5. Baby furniture

   a. A crib and dresser should be purchased before delivery

   b. It is a law that the baby leave the hospital in a safety-approved car seat

6. Baby's sex

   a. During the ultrasound examination, we can often determine the fetal sex by looking for a penis or scrotum

   b. A procedure (amniocentesis) to measure hormone levels or look at genetic chromosomes is expensive and potentially hazardous

V. Outpatient Laboratory Tests

A. Routine labs

1. At initial prenatal visit: blood type, blood Rh and antibody screen, complete blood count, rubella titer, urinalysis, urine cultures, serologic test for syphilis (VDRL or RPR), pap smear, hepatitis B surface antigen (HB_sAg)

2. At the beginning of the third trimester (24-28 weeks): complete blood count, 1-hour post 50 gm glucola glucose determination (diabetes screen), and antibody screen (if Rh negative and unsensitized)

B. Maternal serum alpha-fetoprotein (MSAFP) screening should be discussed and, if the patient desires, should be undertaken between the 15th and 20th weeks

C. Indications for special tests during pregnancy

Special Test	Indications
Gonorrhea culture	Prior veneral infection, vaginitis, drug abuser, adolescent
Clean-catch urine for culture	Patients with consecutively positive abnormal screening urines, symptoms strongly suggestive or urinary tract infection, history of renal disease
Herpes culture	Vulvar lesion, prior infection, recent exposure
HIV antibody	Patients at increased risk i.e., intravenous drug abusers, prostitutes, hemophiliacs, and sexual partners at increased risk because of the above factors or homosexual activity
Shielded chest x-ray	Positive tuberculin skin test, significant past or present respiratory or cardiac illness
Ultrasound	Uncertain menstrual dates, uterine size and dates disparity, prior cesarean section, medical or obstetric complications, poor obstetric history
Diabetes screen (before 24th week)	Family history of diabetes, prior macrosomic fetus, poor obstetric history, persistent glycosuria, suspected polyhydramnios, maternal age 35 or older, obesity, recurrent moniliasis, prior anomalous infant
Hemoglobin A_{1C}	Maternal diabetes or prior macrosomic infant
Rubella titer (later in pregnancy)	If prior titer was 1:8-1:16 or suspected exposure to rubella if titer less than 1:16
Paternal blood typing	Rh negative mother-to-be; uncertainty of father-to-be

NORMAL AND ABNORMAL LABOR

I. Definition of Labor

A. Adequate uterine contractions leading to progressive cervical change and descent of the fetus

B. True vs. false labor

True Labor	False Labor
Back and abdominal discomfort	Lower abdominal discomfort
No relief from sedation	Relief from sedation
Intensity increasing	Intensity unchanged
Regular intervals, gradually increasing	Irregular intervals and duration
Cervical dilation occurs	No cervical dilation

II. Uterine Contraction Patterns

	Frequency	Duration	Indentibility of uterus	Uterine pressure change
Adequate	q 2-3 minutes	45-60 sec	None	> 50 mm Hg
Fair	q 4-5 min	30-45 sec	Slight	20-49 mm Hg
Poor	q 6+ min	< 30 sec	Easy	< 20 mm Hg

III. Assessment of the Fetus

A. Lie - relationship of the long axis (spine) of the fetus to that of the mother (either longitudinal, transverse or oblique)

B. Presentation - part of the fetus that is nearest the pelvic inlet (felt by cervical exam); for example - cephalic or breech

C. Position - relationship between a reference point on the fetal presenting part and the maternal pelvis. The occiput is used in cephalic, the sacrum in breech and the chin in face presentations

IV. Evaluation of Cervix

A. Dilation - describes the degree of opening of the cervical os. Undilated (closed) to complete (10 cm)

B. Effacement - describes the process of thinning. Changes from full thickness (0% effaced) to complete (100% effaced) with labor

C.   Station - describes the relationship between the fetal presenting part and the ischial spines. Zero station is at the level of the spines; example 1 cm above is -1, 2 cm below is +2.

V.   Stages of Labor

A.   First Stage
  1.   From the onset of true labor to complete dilation of the cervix
  2.   Six to 16 hours in a nulliparous and 2 to 10 hours in a multipara patient
  3   Phases
      a.   Latent: 0-3 cm dilation; time for the cervix to become favorable (softer, more effaced)
      b.   Active: 4-10 cm dilation

B.   Second Stage
  1.   From complete dilation of the cervix to birth of the infant
  2.   30 minutes to 3 hours in a nulliparous and 5 to 30 minutes in multipara patient
  3.   The median duration is slightly under 20 minutes in multiparas, and just under 50 minutes for primigravidas

C.   Third Stage
  1.   From the birth of the infant to delivery of the placenta
  2.   5- to 30 minutes

D.   Labor curve

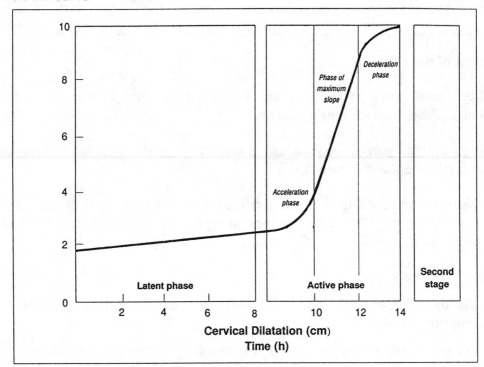

Labor curve adapted from Friedman, 1978.

VI. Abnormal Labor

A. Patterns of abnormal labor

Labor Pattern	Nulligravida	Multiparous	Treatment
Prolonged latent phase	>20 h	> 14 h	Rest or oxytocin

Protraction disorders
   Dilatation
 	
   Descent
	< 1.2 cm/h
	
	< 1.0 cm/h
		<1.5 cm/h
		
		< 2.0 cm/h
			Oxytocin, if contractions are in-adequate

Arrest disorders
   Dilatation
 	
   Descent
	>2 h
	
	>1 h
		>2 h
		
		>1 h
			Oxytocin, if contractions are inadequate
			Forceps, vacuum, or cesarean delivery

B. Evaluate the "P's"
   1. Passenger - is the baby abnormally positioned? large baby?
   2. Passage - adequate pelvis for delivery?
   3. Powers - is contraction pattern adequate?

C. Complications
   1. Maternal
      a. Discomfort, exhaustion, dehydration, uterine rupture
   2. Fetal
      a. Excess molding of head
      b. reduced reserve leading to a worrisome fetal heart rate pattern suggesting "stress" or " distress"

INTRAPARTUM FETAL HEART RATE MONITORING

I. **Clinical Significance**

    A. Electronic fetal heart rate (FHR) monitoring was introduced in the early 1970's after studies supported the existence of a correlation between patterns of fetal heart rate and signs of fetal hypoxia - intrapartum fetal death, fetal blood pH and Apgar scores.

        1. It was hoped that by carefully monitoring intrapartum events, subsequent neurologic damage could be prevented.

    B. Since 1976, there have been several prospective, randomized trials of electronic fetal monitoring.

        1. None of these studies found decreases in the rates of intrapartum death, low Apgar scores, or fetal acidosis when compared to intermittent auscultation

    C. Several studies have shown no change or even a slight increase in the incidence of cerebral palsy in the past 25 years.

    D. Despite its limitations, electronic FHR monitoring is a valuable technique for fetal evaluation.

II. **Uterine Activity Monitoring**

    A. Allows for more accurate interpretation of certain FHR patterns which coincide with contractions

    B. External monitoring

        1. Tocodynamometer
           a. Essentially a weight with a centrally placed pressure-sensitive button which is strapped to the abdominal wall

        2. Monitors contraction frequency but not intensity

    C. Internal monitoring

        1. Membranes must be ruptured

        2. Uses catheters having a pressure-sensing device in tips which are placed in the amniotic cavity.

        3. Accurately monitors frequency, duration, and strength of contractions.
           a. Montevideo unit = average intensity mm Hg x frequency over 10 minutes. Adequate is > 200 montevideo units
           b. Generally, contraction strength = 50 mm Hg and occurring every 3 minutes are considered adequate.

III. Baseline Fetal Heart Rate

    A.   Normal heart rate

        1.   Modulated by the autonomic nervous system of the fetus

        2.   Normal range from 120-160 beats per minutes (bpm)

        3.   Normal range rate decreases slightly with gestational age (155 bpm at 20 weeks; 140 bpm at term)

        4.   Fetal tachycardia
            a.   Baseline heart rate in excess of 160 bpm
            b.   Seen in some cases of fetal asphyxia but not by itself (Normal FHR variability is reassuring).
            c.   Nonasphyxial causes: maternal fever (chorioamnionitis), drugs, parasympatholytic (atropine/vistaril), B-sympathomimetic (terbutaline), tachyarrhythmias (e.g. SVT), fetal anemia/fetal heart failure

        5.   Fetal bradycardia
            a.   Baseline under 120 bpm
            b.   An initial response of the normal fetus to acute hypoxia or asphyxia
            c.   "Moderate bradycardia" (100-120 bpm) with normal variability is usually well-tolerated
            d.   Congenital heart block should be considered.

    B.   Fetal heart rate variability

        1.   Definition and significance
            a.   The most important characteristic in predicting status of the fetus at any given point
            b.   Caused by normal variance in intervals of consecutive cardiac cycles
            c.   Normal values are plus/minus 2 to 3 bpm.
            d.   Irregularity of fetal heart rate baseline, generally at a frequency of 3-5 cycles/minute. Amplitude range greater than 6 bpm
            e.   In the presence of normal variability, no matter what other FHR patterns may be present, fetuses are believed to not be suffering cerebral tissue asphyxia, because they have been able to centralize the available oxygen and compensate physiologically.

        2.   Causes of decrease beat-to-beat variability
            a.   Hypoxia/acidosis
            b.   Drugs (morphine, meperidine, Stadol, MgSO4)
            c.   Fetal sleep cycles
            d.   Congenital anomalies
            e.   Extreme prematurity
            f.   Fetal tachycardia

IV. Periodic FHR Changes

A. Transient heart rate accelerations or decelerations of brief duration with return to the original baseline heart rate.

B. Early decelerations

1. Uniformly shaped and of slow onset and slow return to baseline

2. Begin early in contraction cycle, nadir at peak of contraction, return to baseline before completion of the contraction

3. Generally seen in active phase of labor (4-7 cm of dilation)

4. Thought to be caused by fetal head compression

5. Innocuous FHR pattern

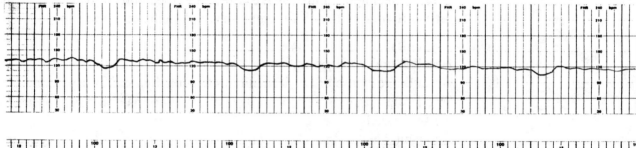

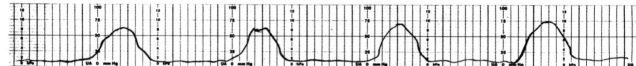

C. Late decelerations

1. Smooth in configuration

2. Onset often 30 sec or more after the onset of the contraction (late)

3. The trough occurs well after contraction peak and usually returns to baseline after the contraction is over

4. Thought to be due to uteroplacental insufficiency - vagally mediated and resulting from fetal hypoxia

5. Persistent late decelerations are significant and potentially ominous; especially with loss of variability.

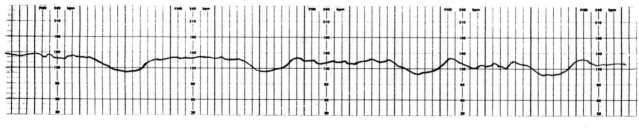

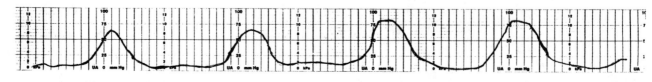

D. Variable decelerations

    1. Variable in duration, intensity and timing relative to uterine contractions

    2. Abrupt in onset and return to baseline

    3. Result of umbilical cord compression

    4. Described as severe when below 60 bpm, 60 bpm below baseline FHR, and > 60 seconds in duration

    5. Most common type of deceleration

    6. Reassuring if rapid return to baseline, normal beat-to-beat variability, not severe and not persistent

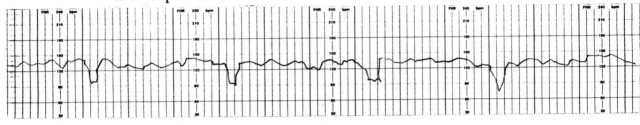

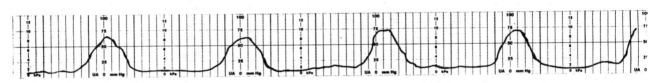

E. Accelerations

    1. Occur most commonly in the antepartum period, early labor, and association with variable decelerations

    2. Associated with fetal movement or uterine contractions

    3. Another cause of partial umbilical cord occlusion

    4. Reassuring

    5. Accelerations with intrapartum pelvic examinations reflect normal fetal scalp pH

V. Medical Management

A. Late decelerations

    1. Place patient on side

    2. Administer O_2 (100%) by tight face mask

    3. Discontinue any oxytocin

    4. Treatment

        a. Appropriate position change

        b. IV hydration

        c. Reserve pharmacologic pressor treatment (ephedrine) for severe or unresponsive hypotension due to conduction anesthesia

        d. Correct any hypertension

B.   Repetitive severe variable decelerations

1.   Change position to where FHR pattern is the most improved (Trendelenburg is often helpful

2.   Discontinue any oxytocin

3.   Check by vaginal examination for cord prolapse or imminent delivery

4.   Administer 100% O_2 by tight face mask

5.   Consider therapeutic amnioinfusion

ANESTHESIA/ANALGESIA IN OBSTETRICS

I.   **Types**

    A.   Local anesthesia
        1.   Subcutaneous injection usually in perineum for episiotomy

    B.   Pudendal
        1.   Analgesia for the perineum
        2.   Short administration to delivery interval
        3.   Easy to administer
        4.   Large drug doses required
        5.   Retroposes and subgluteal abscesses have occurred

    C.   Paracervical
        1.   For active labor only
        2.   No perineal analgesia
        3.   Fetal bradycardia risk limits use
        4.   Use lidocaine 1%

    D.   Spinal (saddle block)
        1.   For delivery
        2.   Requires small dosage of local anesthetic
        3.   May get post-spinal headache
        4.   May produce hypotension due to sympathetic block causing vasodilation
        5.   Frequently used for scheduled Cesarean section
        6.   May create poor motor function and pushing ability

    E.   Lumbar epidural
        1.   Effects innervation of uterus for relief during labor.
        2.   Can be continuously infused for constant level of relief.
        3.   Can give narcotics via epidural.
        4.   Provides sympathetic block which leads to peripheral vasodilation and hypotension. This may cause transient fetal bradycardia.
        5.   May slow early labor (< 5 cm).
        6.   Transient decrease in uterine activity after injection of drug.
        7.   May prolong second stage.
        8.   Contraindications include CNS disease, infection at placement site, coagulopathy, precipitate labor, extreme obesity, severe anemia, sepsis, fetal distress and blood pressure abnormalities.

    F.   General anesthesia
        1.   For cesarean deliveries, especially emergent cases.

II.   **Pain Pathways**

    A.   T-10 through L-1 from uterus/cervix

    B.   S-2 through S-4 from vagina and perineum.

III.   **General Considerations**

    A.   Obstetric anesthesia affects two people

    B.   Many cases are emergencies with suboptimally prepared patients (full stomachs).

    C.   Be aware of medical conditions each patient may have i.e. heart disease, diabetes, asthma.

    D.   Be aware of normal physiological changes of pregnancy involving various systems such as cardiovascular, respiratory, gastrointestinal, etc.

VAGINAL DELIVERY AND OPERATIVE OBSTETRICS

I. **Mechanisms of Labor**

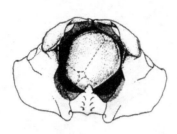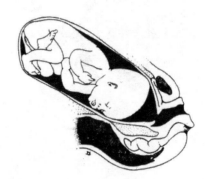

A. Onset of labor.

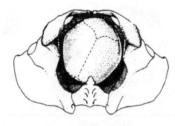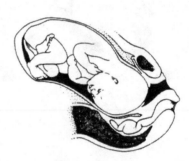

B. Descent and flexion.

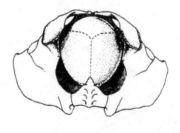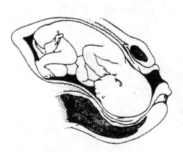

C. Internal rotation: LOA to OA.

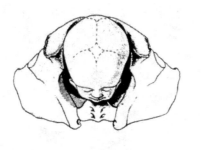
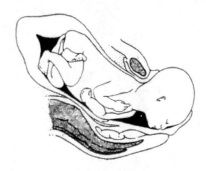

D. Extension.

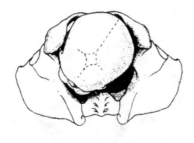
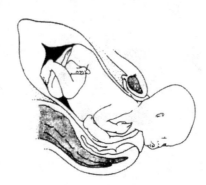

E. Restitution: OA to LOA.

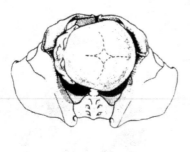
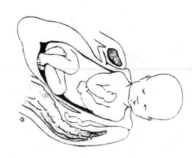

F. External rotation: LOA to LOT.

From: Oxorn-Foote, <u>Human Labor</u> & <u>Birth</u>, 5th ed., Appleton-Century-Crofts, 1986

II. Checklist for Vaginal Delivery

    A.   The following steps are to be taken in sequential order during the delivery process
        1.   Allow for crowning of fetal head
        2.   Cut episiotomy (if necessary) with special scissors
        3.   Control delivery of head
        4.   Allow for restitution & external rotation of head
        5.   Suction upper airways (mouth and nares)
        6.   Apply hands to head and mandible
        7.   Downward (45°) traction and delivery of anterior shoulder
        8.   Upward traction (45°) with delivery of posterior shoulder
        9.   Control delivery of body
        10.   Hold baby on forearm at level of perineum
        11.   Doubly clamp and incise umbilical cord
        12.   Dry baby with towel, show to parents, and place in radiant heater or wrap in blanket
        13.   Gentle traction on cord and elevate uterus (Brandt-andrews maneuver)
        14.   Deliver placenta in basin and inspect placenta and membranes
        15.   Massage atonic uterus
        16.   Inspect perineum and vaginal vault using hand and sponged ring forceps
        17   Pitocin to help uterus contract

III. Operative Obstetrics

    A.   Episiotomy
        1.   Most common surgery
        2.   Usually midline (rather than mediolateral) of lower third of posterior vagina and upper perineum
        3.   May extend into anus (third degree perineal tear) or anus and rectum (fourth degree tear)
        4.   Repair of midline episiotomy

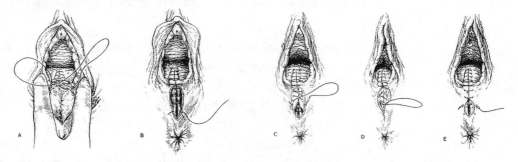

From: Williams Obstetrics, 19th ed., Appleton & Lange 1993

B.   Forceps/Vacuum

    1.   Indications

        a.   Failure to descend during second stage from maternal exhaustion of epidural analgesia

        b.   Abnormal fetal heart rate pattern such as repetitive FHR variable decelerations or bradycardia

    2.   Prerequisite before application

        a.   Cervix fully dilated

        b.   Ruptured membranes

        c.   Position and station of fetal known and engaged

        d.   Anesthesia adequate for maternal comfort

        e.   Maternal pelvis found appropriate

    3.   Classification

        a.   *Outlet forceps*: The fetal skull has reached the perineal floor, the scalp is visible between contractions, the sagittal suture is in the anteroposterior diameter or in the right or left occiput anterior or posterior position, but not more than 45° from the midline.

        b.   *Low forceps*: The leading edge of the skull is station +2 or more. Rotations are divided into 45° or less and more than 45°.

        c.   *Midforceps*: The head is engaged but the leading edge of the skull is above +2 station.

    4   Advantages

        a   Forceps: better traction allows for rotation

        b.   Vacuum: no forceps marks, limited traction allowed

C.   Cesarean section

    1.   National average 20-25% (<5% in 1965); approximately one-third are repeat surgeries

    2.   Usually Pfannenstiel ("bikini" or low transverse) skin incision with low transverse uterine incision

        a.   For cosmetic effect and less chance of uterine rupture

        b.   Vertical incisions allow for more space (i.e. delivery of twins)

    3.   Indications

        a.   Failure to progress from inadequate descent or cervical dilation from fetopelvic disproportion

        b.   Suspected fetal distress according to abnormal fetal heart rate pattern. May be accompanied by meconium, fetal scalp pH < 7.20, lack of heart rate accelerations to tactile or vibroacoustic stimulation

        c.   Fetal malpresentation/mid position such as transverse lie, breech, persistent occiput posterior (fully flexed neck) transverse arrest persistent (left or right occiput transverse position) and face (mentum posterior)

        d.   Repeat cesarean section accounts for one-third of all cesarean sections

    e.   Rapidly deteriorating maternal disorder (severe preeclampsia) with unfavorable cervix

    f.   Other: placenta previa, large placental abruption, active genital herpes infection, twins (usually if malpresentation, monoamniotic, very premature), space occupying fetal anomaly hydrocephaly, meningomyelocele, abdominal wall defect; and umbilical cord prolapse

4.   Minimizing risks
    a.   Prophylactic antibiotics
    b.   Epidural rather than general anesthesia
    c.   Meticulous hemostasis
    d.   Minimize tissue injury or handling

5.   Complications
    a.   Operative: injury to bowel and bladder, broad ligament hematoma, excess hemorrhage
    b.   Anesthesia: incomplete epidural block, difficulty with intubation and extubation, sedation of fetus, and vomiting and aspiration
    c.   Postoperative: anemia, postpartum fever, delay of recovery, prolonged hospitalization

6.   Vaginal birth after cesarean section (VBAC)
    a.   Childbirth preparation
    b.   Analgesia: none or minimal amount encouraged
    c.   Precautions during labor: continuous fetal heart rate and uterine activity monitoring
    d.   Sterilization desired: does not contraindicate VBAC; if cesarean necessary, should discuss sterilization beforehand
    e.   Previous scar formation; discuss removal of skin scar, increased risk of adhesions with present or future surgeries
    f.   Hospital capabilities: requires anesthesia and operating room crew to be aware and available, limitations in many rural communities
    g.   Contraindicated by prior classical incision. recurrent fetopelvic disproportion or accompanying complication requiring cesarean section
    i.   Incision types

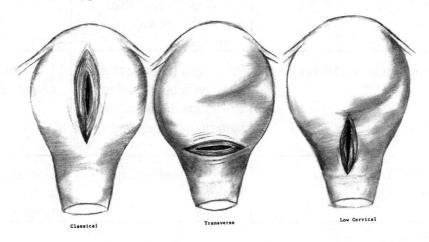

      Classical   Transverse   Low Cervical

OBSTETRIC PROCEDURES

	Indications	Complications
I.Dilation and Curettage (D&C)		
A. Early	Incomplete, missed, or elective abortion	Uterine perforation; incomplete removal of conceptus; endomyometritis, Rh isoimmunization, hemorrhage
B. Postpartum	Hemorrhage from suspected retained placental fragments	Same as above
II. Amniocentesis		
A. Genetic (14-18 weeks)	Increased risk of chromosomal abnormality (advanced maternal age, low MSAFP, prior affected child, X-linked disease)	Hemorrhage from placenta; Rh isoimmunization; injury to fetus or umbilical cord; stillbirth (likely no increased risk using ultrasound guidance)
	Increased risk of open neural tube defect (for AFP and acetylcholinesterase level)	
	Increased risk of inborn error of metabolism	
B. Nongenetic	Fetal lung maturity (L/S ratio, PG testing; Intra-amniotic infection screening (gram stain culture)	Same as above
III. Cervical Cerclage	A previously suspected incompetent cervix (painless cervical dilation during the second trimester)	Localized infection and hemorrhage; premature labor
IV. Forceps/Vacuum Delivery	Prolonged second stage with ineffective pushing; worrisome fetal heart rate pattern during second stage	Misapplication; trauma to head; vaginal/perineal tears
V. Newborn Circumcision	Cosmetic and perhaps hygiene reasons	Inadequate hemostasis; localized infection; excess of imprecise removal of skin

IMMEDIATE CARE OF THE NEWBORN

I. Anticipated Difficulties

A. Intrapartum signs
1. Risk factors: meconium, abnormal fetal heart rate pattern, fetal growth problems
2. Need for operative delivery (forceps, cesarean)?
3. Gestational age: very premature, postdate
4. Fetal malpresentation

B. Birth
1. Search for external anomalies
2. Assign Apgar scores at 1 and 5 minutes

Sign	0 Points	1 Point	2 Points
Heart rate	Absent	Under 100	Over 100
Respiratory effort	Absent	Slow-irregular	Good crying
Muscle tone	limp	flexion of extremities	Active Motion
Reflex irritability; response to catheter in nostril	No response	Grimace	Cough or sneeze
Color	blue-white	body pink, extremities blue	completely pink

II. Immediate Care

A. Place under radiant heater

B. Suction trachea if meconium

C. Dry thoroughly

D. Position with head down

E. Suction mouth, then nose

F. Provide tactile stimulation

III. Resuscitation and Considerations

A. Evaluate respirations
1. None or gasping
   a. Positive pressure ventilation (PPV) with 100% oxygen (15-30 secs)
2. Spontaneous
   a. Evaluate color and provide oxygen if cyanosis or acrocyanosis
3. Monitor heart rate at same time

B. Evaluate heart rate
1. If below 60:
   a. Continue ventilation
   b. Chest compressions
   c. Initiate medication (sodium bicarbonate, epinephrine)below 80 after 30 seconds, PPV with 100% oxygen and chest compression
2. If 60 - 100
   a. Heart rate not increasing - continue ventilation, chest compressions
   b. Heart rate increasing - continue ventilation
3. If above 100
   a. Watch for spontaneous respirations
   b. Discontinue ventilation
4. Evaluate for color
   a. Pink or peripheral cyanosis - observe and monitor

IV. Birthweight and Gestational Age

A. Physical findings and gestational age
1. Examine skin, lanugo, vernix, sole creases, breast tissue, ear shape and cartilage, genitalia (male: testes and rugae, female: labia), and posture

B.. Birthweight
1. Influences
   a. Multiparous or male: slight increase
   b. African-American: slight decrease

2. Assign percentile for gestational age
   a. Appropriate for gestational age (AGA): > 10% - < 90%
   b. Small for gestational age (SGA): ≤ 10%
   c. Severe: ≤ 5%; mild:6-10%

3. Symmetric
   a. small all over
   b. Onset in early gestation
   c. Causes: constitutional, chromosome, chronic infection, chronic maternal vascular disorder

4. Asymmetric
   a. "Head sparing", head appropriately sized but abdomen and subcutaneous skin small
   b. Onset in later gestation
   c. Causes: hypertension, placental dysfunction, smoking

5. Large for gestational age (LGA): ≥ 90%
   a. Causes: constitutional, diabetes, edema
   b. "Cherub" body (fat all around, offspring of a diabetic) versus constitutionally long and well-proportioned infant

V. Observation

    A. Physical findings
        1. Rapid respiratory rate (>65), apnea, cyanotic
        2. Abdominal distention, poor feeding, vomiting
        3. Lethargy, irritability, jitteriness
        4. Heart rate < 80 or > 200 bpm
        5. Axillary temperature $< 36.3°$ C or $\geq 38°$ C

    B. Laboratories
        1. Glucose Chemstrip
            a. To be performed on infants of diabetic mother, LGA or SGA infant, jitteriness, or low 5-min Apgar
            b. If 0-20 mg%, give 2 ml/kg DIOW IV over 5 min
                If 20-40 mg%, give 10 ml/kg of DIOW and formula

        2. Hematocrit: infants of diabetic, suspected sepsis, LGA or SGA infant, jitteriness, prethoric appearance

        3. Serum calcium: to infant of diabetic, LGA or SGA infant, jitteriness

        4. VDRL: all infants

        5. Blood type and direct Coombs: mother who is Rh(-), unsensitized

        6. Urine drug serum: mother with substance abuse or no prenatal care, jitteriness, floppy

        7. Bilirubin: if jaundice

        8. PKU: all infants

        9. T4/TSH:requires prompt treatment if phenylketonuria exists

VI. Routine Care

    A. Medications

Medication	Condition to Treat
Oxygen	Depressed respirations
Naloxone	Excess maternal narcotics
Vitamin K	Deficiency which would impact on clotting factor synthesis
Tetracycline ophthalmalgic ointment	Safeguard against or treat against gonorrhea or chlamydia conjunctivitis
Triple dye	Promote healing of umbilical cord
Dextrose	Hypoglycemia

B.   Feedings
    1.   Initially sterile water to see if difficulty feeding
    2.   Ad lib bottle or breast feeding
        a.   Often takes 24 hours
        b.   Within 4 hours of birth
        c.   Maximum of 6 hours between feedings
        d.   Bottle feeding; 150-200 ml/kg/d if no breast feeding; 75 ml/kg/d if breast feeding

C.   Stools and Urine
    1.   Absent?
    2.   Blood?

D.   Vital signs: observe for fever, tachypnea

E.   Other
    1.   Daily weights - anticipate 5-10% loss
    2.   Neurobehavioral testing - Dubowitz
    3.   Jaundice - Sclera, skin
    4.   Circumcision if desired for males
    4.   Bathing instructions
    5.   Parent education on routine care and return clinic visit

POSTPARTUM CARE

I. Physiologic Changes

A. Postpartum period (puerperium) is the 6-week period after delivery
    1. Many changes return to normal in 2 weeks after delivery

B. Uterus
    1. Involution
        a. Fundus at umbilicus shortly after delivery, at symphysis by 2 weeks, and nonpregnant size by 6 weeks
        b. More rapid with breast feeding
    2. Discharge ("lochia")
        a. Blood in first 3 days: may be present for several weeks in small amounts
        b. Brownish clear by end of first week

C. Cervix
    1. Regains shape within hours
    2. External os appears transverse and fish-mouthed

D. Ovaries
    1. Ovulation may occur in 2 weeks if delivery $\leq$ 20 weeks or 4 weeks if delivery at term
    2. Remains delayed or suppressed if the presence of elevated prolactin levels in lactating women

E. Cardiovascular
    1. Previously elevated pulse rate, and cardiac output returns to normal within hours
    2. Expanded intravascular volume is affected by shift in fluids from extracellular space and increased diuresis

F. Blood count
    1. Anemia frequently becomes apparent, necessitating a need for iron supplementation
    2. Leukocytosis is common as part of the normal healing process

II. Routine Care

A. Discharge from hospital
    1. After an uncomplicated delivery is usually the next day after a vaginal delivery or second full postoperative day

B. Routine observation
    1. Examine for anemia
        a. Signs: tachycardia, orthostatic hypotension, hematocrit, excess lochia, clots passed

      b.   Complete blood count on first postpartum day

2. Follow for fever
   a. If present, consider atelectasis, endomyometritis, wound, urinary tract infection, "flu-like" illness

3. Attempt to minimize thrombophlebitis
   a. Early ambulation
   b. Observe for signs of deep venous thrombophlebitis

4. Encourage maternal-infant bonding
   a. Breast feeding assistance
   b. Rooming-in: daytime vs. all day
   c. Private rooms

5. Provide analgesia
   a. Postoperative
      1. Sites: incision, abdominal muscle stretching, uterine cramping
      2. Patient controlled analgesia vs. intramuscular narcotics
   b. Vaginal delivery
      1. Site: episiotomy or perineal tears and uterine cramping
      2. Usual relief from oral prostaglandin synthetase inhibitor, acetaminophen, or codeine/hydrocodone

6. Lactation
   a. Often attempted and should be encouraged
   b. May cause more rapid uterine involution, vaginal dryness, and more rapid weight loss
   c. Rich source of immunoglobulins
   d. Nursing service is often a major patient education asset
   e. Ovulation and menses are less frequent and predictable
   f. Most medications cross into breast milk but in very low concentrations
   g. Nonpharmacologic suppression: cold compresses, tight fitting bra, avoid stimulation
   h.. Drug-induced suppressor - bromocriptine (Parlodel)
      1. Does not need to be routinely prescribed
      2. Avoid if hypertension (risk of cardiovascular accident?)

7. Provide select immunotherapy
   a. Anti D immune globulin (RhoGAM®) if mother is D negative and infant positive
   b. Rubella vaccine if mother is nonimmune

III. Counseling

A. Care of infant
   1. State law requires that each infant receive silver nitrate, erythromycin, or tetracycline in its eyes to guard against gonorrhea and chlamydia conjunctivitis
   2. Encourage a pediatrician or family physician to be chosen beforehand

3. It is not necessary for that doctor to attend the delivery or see the baby shortly after delivery but may be desirable

4. The baby's first visit should be scheduled usually within the first month (usually within two weeks)after delivery

5. It is a law in Oklahoma that the baby leave the hospital in a safety-approved car seat

B. Contraception

1. Foam and condoms are often recommended until return to clinic

   a. Most persons are sexually active until return to clinic but still require safeguards

2. Consider any medical disorders, prior contraception success/failures, desire for future childbearing or sterilization (patient vs. spouse) when selecting form of contraception

C. Anxiety and depression

1. Common in variable degrees for both new mother and father

2. Risk factors: marital discord, prior postpartum problems, known psychiatric illness, habitual abortion or stillbirth, anomalous infant, prematurity, antepartum anxiety or depression

3. Hormones or hereditary etiologies are unclear but require attention

4. Commonly adjustment problems which are temporary (first month) if no other risk factors

   a. "Postpartum blues"

   b. May not be apparent until after discharge

   c. Watch for signs of inability to experience pleasure or happiness

5. Encourage patients to participate actively in childbirth preparation and care of infant

6. More extreme or prolonged signs of anxiety or depression require further counselling and perhaps medication

D. Exercise

1. To promote support of the abdominal muscles

2. May begin immediately after hospital discharge

3. Overstrenuous exercise is to be discouraged, during the initial 2 weeks

4. After a cesarean section, strenuous exercises other than walking are to be avoided until return to the office in usually 2 weeks after delivery

E. Postpartum office visit

1. Usually at 4-6 weeks if uncomplicated vaginal delivery and at 2 and 6 weeks postoperatively

2. Search for interactions of newborn with family, any adjustment difficulty, resumption of coitus, contraception, resumption of work and activities

3. Examine for blood pressure elevations, breast masses or tenderness, uterine size, anemia

4. Obtain pap smear and screen for diabetes if previously gestational-onset diabetic

5. Review progress of recent pregnancy and discuss ramifications on future childbearing

6. Continue to encourage healthy habits
   a. Proper nutrition, regular exercise, avoid smoking and other substance abuse, and adequate rest

POSTPARTUM STERILIZATION

I. Patient Profile

A. Two or more healthy children

B. At least 21 years old

C. May have active medical disorder (diabetes, hypertension) in which nonpermanent contraception is a problem

II. Prenatal Counseling

A. Failure rate (per 100 year use)

1.	None				90
2.	Nonpermanent contraception				
	a.	Natural, rhythm			15-45
	b.	Hormonal suppression			
		1)	Oral contraceptives		<1-2
		2)	Norplant		<1-3
		3)	Depo Provera		<1-3
	c.	Barrier			
		1)	Foam, gel		15-35
		2)	Foam & condoms		5-15
		3)	Diaphragm (with spermicide)		10-20
	d.	Intrauterine device			2-4
3.	Permanent contraception				
	a.	Vasectomy			1
	b.	Postpartum bilateral tubal ligation			0.2
	c.	Laparoscopic fulguration, clip, fallope ring			0.2

B. Signed permit with explanation of surgery

III. Preoperative Checklist

A. Infant and patient doing well

B. Understands risks and other forms of contraception

C. Understands option of delaying surgery and performing laparoscopic procedure

D. Negative pap smear

E. Permit signed and on chart

IV. Procedures

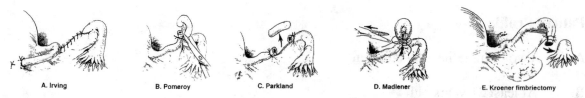

A. Irving   B. Pomeroy   C. Parkland   D. Madlener   E. Kroener fimbriectomy

From: <u>Williams</u> <u>Obstetrics</u>, 19th ed., Appleton & Lange, 1993

V. Complications

A. Immediate
1. Anesthesia: incomplete, intubation difficulties, aspiration,
2. Infection: incision, intra-abdominal
3. Concealed hemorrhage
4. Injury to bowel

B. Delayed

1. Failed sterilization
   a. Ligated round ligament
   b. Tube recanalized

2. Pelvic pain or menstrual irregularity
   a. Very unlikely attributed to surgery
   b. Probably had before pregnancy

3. Depression

4. Requests reanastomosis

COMMON OBSTETRIC ABBREVIATIONS

History

IUP ------------ Intrauterine pregnancy
LMP----------- Last menstrual period (first day of)
LNMP--------- Last normal menstrual period
EDC, EDD --- Estimated date of confinement (or delivery)
G--------------- Gravida (pregnant woman)
P -------------- Parity
Ab ------------- Abortion
TAb ----------- Therapeutic abortion
EAb ----------- Elective abortion
EGA----------- Estimated Gestational Age

Physical Examination

FH ------------- Fundal height (cm's from symphysis to fundus)
FHT ----------- Fetal heart tones
FHR ----------- Fetal heart rate
EFW ---------- Estimated fetal weight
Cx ------------- Cervix
IUFD---------- Intrauterine fetal death
SB ------------- Stillbirth

Prenatal Labs

GC------------- Gonorrhea
HI-------------- Hemagglutination inhibition (test used to determine rubella Ab titer > 1:8 is
                         protective)
G6PD --------- Glucose-6-phosphate dehydrogenase level
IAS ------------ Irregular antibody screen

Fetal Assessment Tests

FM, FMC----- Fetal movement, fetal movement charting
NST ----------- Passive monitoring (of fetal heart rate accelerations with fetal motion) or nonstress
                         testing
OCT,CST ---- Oxytocin challenge test or contraction stress testing
US, U/S------- Ultrasound
L/S------------- Lecithin-spingomyetin ratio
PG ------------- Phosphatidyl glycerol

Fetal Size and Body Measurements

IUGR---------- Intrauterine growth retardation
SGA----------- Small for gestational age
LGA----------- Large for gestational age
BPD----------- Biparietal diameter
FL ------------- Femur length
AC------------- Abdominal circumference
HC------------- Head circumference

COMMON OBSTETRIC ABBREVIATIONS (Cont'd)

Intrapartum Terms

    L&D----------- Labor and delivery
    ctxn------------ contraction
    pit-------------- Pitocin (synthetic oxytocin)
    BOWI--------- Bag of waters intact
    PROM -------- Premature rupture of membranes
    SROM -------- Spontaneous rupture of membranes
    AROM-------- Artificial rupture of membranes
    SVD----------- Spontaneous vaginal delivery (SCVD   controlled)
    ELF------------ Elective low forceps delivery
    MF------------- Mid forceps delivery
    CS, C/S ------- Cesarean section
    RCS ----------- Repeat cesarean section
    BPS ----------- Bilateral partial salpingectomy

Fetal Positions During Labor

    OA------------- Occiput anterior
    LOA----------- Left OA
    OP ------------- Occiput posterior (plus LOP & ROP)
    LOT ----------- Left occiput transverse (Plus ROT)
    ROA ---------- Right OA

Postpartum Terms

    PP ------------- Postpartum
    pph ------------ Postpartum hemorrhage
    D&C ---------- Dilation and curettage
    PPTL---------- Postpartum tubal ligation
    BTL ----------- Bilateral tubal ligation
    OC------------- Oral contraceptive

ABNORMAL OBSTETRICS

SPONTANEOUS AND ELECTIVE ABORTION

I. **Definition**

    A.   Termination of pregnancy before 20 weeks from the last menstrual period

II. **Incidence**

    A.   Positive sensitive pregnancy test only:- 50% of all pregnancies

    B.   Recognized tissue: 20-25% of all pregnancies
        1.   80% in first 12 weeks

III. **Etiology**

    A.   Chromosomes - 50% (for first trimester)

    B.   Other
        1.   Medical illness (diabetes, collagen vascular disease, hyperthyroidism)
        2.   Infection (listeria, mycoplasma, ureaplasma, toxoplasmosis)
        3.   Advanced maternal or paternal age
        4.   Grand multiparity
        5.   Abnormal placental development
        6.   Uterine defects (septum, bicornuate, leiomyoma)
        7.   More than 3 elective first trimester abortions

IV. **Differential Diagnosis**

	Active Bleeding	Internal Cervical Os	Uterine Size	Therapy
Threatened	Spotting	Closed	= dates	Expectant
Incomplete	Active bleeding	Open	< dates	Dilation and curettage (D&C)
Complete	Minimal	Closed	Nonpregnant	None
Missed	Little or none	Closed	< dates	Dilation & evacuation (D&E)

V. **Diagnostic Tests**

    A.   Ultrasonography
        1.   Transvaginal: see sac at 5 weeks, serum BhCG level $\geq$ 2,000 mIU/ml
        2.   Transabdominal: see sac at 6 weeks; serum BhCG level $\geq$ 5,000 mIU/ml

    B.   Examination of retrieved tissue
        1.   Under low power microscope
        2.   See if floats on water

VI. **Recurrent Abortion -** two consecutive or total of at least three spontaneous abortions

    A.   Further counseling
        1.   Emotional support: alleviate fears of what was done or not done to avoid
        2.   Recurrent risk: after 1 abortion (20%), 2 abortions (25%), 3 abortions (30%)

    B.   Evaluation of parents-to-be (Note: Same as if stillborn infant)
        1.   Parental karyotyping for balanced translocation
        2.   Screen for diabetes, thyroid dysfunction, collagen vascular disease
        3.   Hysterosalpingogram

VII. **Postabortion Therapy**

    A.   Uterine stimulants: oral or intramuscular methylergonovine (Methergine)

    B.   Antibiotics: single oral agent if prolonged or excess bleeding, much uterine manipulation, known genital infection

    C.   Rh immune globulin
        1.   If Rh negative, fetus may have been positive so anti-D Rh immune globulin (RhoGAM) necessary
        2.   MICRhoGAM before 12 weeks

ECTOPIC PREGNANCY

I. Definition

A. Implantation of fertilized ovum outside the uterine cavity
1. Sites: fallopian tube (95%, primarily ampulla), cervix, ovary, bowel, peritoneum

II. Incidence and Risk Factors

A. 1 in every 66 intrauterine pregnancies

B. Risk factors: prior salpingitis, older maternal age (35-44 yo), ≥ 3 pregnancies, African-American or Hispanic, failed sterilization, prior infertility (possible tubal disease)

III. Differential Diagnosis

Disorder	Symptoms	Physical Findings	Laboratory
Abortion	Pelvic cramping, spotting	Cervix open, enlarged uterus, nontender adnexa	BhCG - positive* Normal wbc Negative Urinalysis US - sac in uterus**
Ectopic pregnancy	Amenorrhea or vaginal spotting and pain (colicky, unilateral), syncope	Cervix closed, small uterus, tender adnexa	BhCG - positive* Normal wbc Negative Urinalysis US - no sac in uterus*
Salpingitis	Recent menses, constant pelvic pain	Fever, tender pelvis, closed cervix	BhCG-negative, Elevated wbc
Ruptured ovarian cyst	Sudden unilateral pain	Tender adnexa, small nontender uterus	BhCG - negative Normal wbc Negative urinalysis
Appendicitis	Unilateral pain, regular menses	Fever, unilateral pain, nontender uterus	BhCG - negative Elevated wbc Negative urinalysis
Ureterolithiasis	Unilateral pelvic and flank pain; regular menses	Flank pain, afebrile (unless pyelonephritis)	BhCG-negative Normal wbc Hematuria

* A quantitative BhCG early in pregnancy should increase by at least 66% in 48 hours with a normal intrauterine pregnancy

** Should see intrauterine sac if BhCG > 2,000 IU/ml using transvaginal scan or > 6,000 IU/ml using transabdominal scan

IV. Risks

    A.   Maternal death
        1.   From hemorrhage
        2.   < 1 per 1,000 cases

    B.   Co-existing intrauterine pregnancy
        1.   1 in 8,000-30,000 pregnancies

    C.   Future pregnancy
        1.   Still favorable for intrauterine pregnancy
        2.   Reassess risk factors
        3.   Screen early in gestation(BhCG, pelvic ultrasound)

    D.   Abdominal pregnancy
        1.   10-30% fetal survival

        2.   If diagnose early, clamp cord, remove fetus, and retained placenta for subsequent resorption
            a.   Follow serum BhCG levels
            b.   Methotrexate, a folic acid antagonist, is commonly used to suppress placenta

    E.   Rh negative, unsensitized mothers; should receive Rh immune globulin

V. Evaluation

    A.   Menstrual history

    B.   Examination
        1.   Bleeding
        2.   Mass
        3.   Tenderness

    C.   Ultrasound
        1.   Localize pregnancy
        2.   Find adnexal complex
        3.   See blood in cul-de-sac

    D.   Culdocentesis - use spinal needle to enter cul-de-sac for posterior vaginal fornix to retrieve fluid
        1.   Non-clotting blood indicates intraperitoneal bleeding
        2.   Pus indicates pelvic/abdominal infection
        3.   Straw colored fluid - normal peritoneal fluid
        4.   No fluid obtained is non-diagnostic

    E.   Laporascopy - to diagnose

VI. Management

A. Surgery
1. Diagnostic laporascopy
   a. If small unruptured tube, perform linear salpingostomy
   b. If larger or ruptured tube, perform segmental resection (with reanastomoses later) or salpingectomy

B. Nonsurgical
1. If small and unruptured, consider oral or intramuscular methotrexate and follow serum BhCG levels

PRENATAL GENETIC COUNSELING

I. **Impact on Obstetric Care**

    A. More awareness of fetal structural or certain genetic conditions either early in gestation or before birth
        1. Options: abortion (if early in gestation) or continue pregnancy and deliver at hospital capable of helping newborn
        2. Reassurance if normal findings
        3. Overall risk of major anomalies at birth: 2-4%

    B. Difficult or impossible to predict behavior and cognitive development in infancy and childhood

II. **Counselling Indications**

    A. Environmental hazards
        1. Radiation
            a. Diagnostic
                1. Much less than 5 rads
                2. No added risk
                3. Recommend shielded x-ray anyway
            b. Therapeutic
                1. Rarely seen
                2. Need dosimetry to counsel

        2. Drugs/chemicals
            a. Very few are associated with specific anomalies
            b. Need to know name of medication, dose, duration, gestational age, accompanying medications and illnesses
            c. Less known in humans about pesticide and workplace chemicals. Should avoid or at least allow minimal exposure in well-ventilated area

        3. Infections
            a. Viruses
                1. Cytomegalovirus, rubella, parvovirus, hepatitis
                2. Mother is often asymptomatic
                3. Fetal risks: growth delay, anemia, stillbirth, intracranial calcifications, blindness, impaired hearing
                4. May linger or remain dormant
                5. Unable to eradicate
            b. Bacterial
                1. Gonorrhea, streptococcal, Klebsiella, E. Coli
                2. Direct risk less than virus
                3. Less subtle since mother is usually symptomatic
                4. Antibiotics may eradicate before or after delivery
                5. More of acute, nonlingering problem than viral infection

B.   Prior anomalous infant
1.   Cause is usually multifactorial, polygenic etiology

2.   Recurrence risk of defect (one affected child)

Midline facial cleft	2-4%	Pyloristenosis	3%
Cardiac	2-5%	Renal agenesis	1-3%
Open neural tube	2-4%		
Hydrocephaly	1%		

3.   Assess any underlying medical disorders (diabetes, seizures) and medication

C.   Family history of mental retardation

1.   Common to find indirect family members

2.   Usually no added risk

3.   Inquire about any chromosomal testing (fragile X), inborn errors of metabolism, or abnormalities during pregnancy in question

D.   Advanced maternal age - routine for 35 and older at the time of delivery

E.   Abnormal MSAFP

III.   Genetic Testing

A.   Alpha fetoprotein (AFP)

1.   A fetal-specific glycoprotein manufactured in the yolk sac

2.   Highest concentration in fetal serum but measurable in smaller amounts in maternal serum (transplacental passage) and amniotic fluid (fetal urine)

3.   Best measured in maternal serum (MSAFP) between 15-20 weeks
    a.   Indication
        1.   Routinely offered
        2.   Prior child with open neural tube defect
        3.   Maternal diabetes
        4.   Prior or current pregnancy complications
    b.   Interpretation
        1.   Elevated: open neural tube defect, abdominal wall defect, erroneous dates, stillbirth, twins, abnormal placenta, nephrosis
        2.   Low: chromosomal (especially trisomy 21), erroneous dates
    c.   Further testing
        1.   Targeted ultrasound
        2.   Amniocentesis for AFP, acetylcholinesterase (ACHE), andchromosomes if low MSAFP or persistently elevated MSAFP

B.   Amniocentesis (usually 14-18 weeks)

Test	Indication
Alpha fetoprotein	Elevated MSAFP; prior child with open neural tube defect
Chromosomes	Maternal age $\geq$ 35 years Low MSAFP Prior child with X-linked disease Prior child with chromosomal disorder
Inborn error of metabolism	Prior child with inborn error metabolism

C.   Chorionic villous sampling

     1.   Aspiration of placental tissue transcervically or transabdominally

     2.   Allows for earlier diagnosis (8-12 weeks)

     3.   Risks
          a.   Contaminated cells may lead to mosaicism
          b.   Increased risk of spontaneous abortion (minimal)

D.   Cordocentesis/periumbilical blood sampling - transabdominal sampling of fetal blood through umbilical cord vein

ANTENATAL INFECTIONS

I. **Gonorrhea**

    A.   Incidence 1 - 3 % of pregnant women

    B.   Untreated gonorrhea associated with PROM, preterm labor, peripartum infections, neonatal ophthalmoplegia

    C.   Treatment reduces risk of adverse outcome

II. **Syphilis**

    A.   Incidence 0.1 - 0.3 %

    B.   Associated with stillbirth, congenital anomalies, preterm delivery

    C.   Therapy early in pregnancy reduces risk of adverse outcome

III **Chlamydia**

    A.   Incidence 3 - 15% of women

    B.   Chlamydia most common among low income, nonwhite, unmarried, teenagers

    C.   Women with chlamydia are at increased risk of low birthweight even after controlling for these factors

    D.   Does therapy of chlamydia reduce risk of low birthweight? Evidence is conflicting

IV. **Ureaplasma**

    A.   Incidence 30 - 80 %

    B.   Most common in poor, nonwhite, unmarried women

    C.   After controlling for other factors, no increase in prematurity in Ureaplasma positive women

    D.   Treatment of Ureaplasma does not reduce risk of prematurity

V. **Group B Strep**

    A.   Incidence 10 - 20 % of population

    B.   Group B Strep sepsis more common in premature infants

    C.   GBS chorioamnionitis more common in premature labor

D.   Uncertain if GBS carriage predicts women at risk for preterm labor

E.   Erythromycin therapy of GBS in mid-gestation does not appear to reduce risk of prematurity

F.   Controversy exists over screening for GBS

VI.   Trichomonas

A.   Incidence 3 - 10 %

B.   Evidence that majority of infections are asymptomatic

C.   Trichomonas carriage is associated with an increased risk of low birth weight

D.   Unknown if therapy reduces risk of LBW

VII.   Bacterial Vaginosis

A.   Incidence 15 - 25 %

B.   Associated with low birth weight, intra-amniotic infection, post partum infection

C.   Unknown if therapy will reduce risk of low birth weight

VIII.   Urinary Tract Infection

A.   Significance

1.   Most common complication

2.   Pyelonephritis is most common medical indication for hospitalization in pregnancy

3.   3 - 10% have significant bacteriuria. Of these, 20-30% will develop pyelonephritis if untreated. Treatment reduces incidence to 2-5%

4.   At least two studies have shown association with anemia - and therapy prevented development of anemia

5.   Controversial aspects
a.   Prematurity
b.   Hypertension
c.   Subsequent renal function

B.   Diagnosis

1.   Culture - Kass showed that $> 10^5$/ml of a single organism represented infection 85% of the time, on two consecutive mornings - 95%, on three consecutive mornings - $> 99\%$.

2. Microscopic exam of urine
   a. WBC - Very misleading
      40% with + culture have no pyuria
      40% with > 20 WBC/HPF have - culture
   b. Bacteria
      Some authors report 80 -90% correlation, others < 50.

3. Symptoms
   a. 50% of women with frequency and dysuria have - culture
   b. 95% of women with fever, flank pain and dysuria have + culture
   c. 3 - 5% of pregnant women have asymptomatic bacteriuria

4. Chemical tests
   a. Griess (Nitrite)
      1. > 99% specific
      2. ~ 90% sensitive on first void specimen
      3. ~ 40% sensitive on random specimen
   b. Uriglox (Glucose)
      1. ~ 95% correlation on first void
      2. ~ 50-60% on random

C. Treatment

1. 75% respond to single course of antibiotics ampicillin, Macrodantin, cephalosporin. 85% respond to Bactrim, but ? fetal effects

2. ~ 25% will have recurrent infection

3. Those with recurrence - retreat, then give Macrodantin 50 - 100 mg h.s. for remainder of pregnancy

4. For chronic suppression - Mandelamine drug of choice. pH urine must be < 6. May require up to 4 g ascorbic acid qd

IX. Herpesvirus Hominus Type II

A. Questioned association with abortion

B. Neonatal infection
   1. 50% of infants develop neonatal herpes and 50% of these die or are seriously damaged
   2. Risk substantially reduced by Cesarean section

X. Congenital Infections

A. Rubella

   1. 10-20% of mothers are not immune

   2. Titer > 1:8 shows immunity

3. Diagnosis of recent infection
   a. HAI antibodies
   b. CF antibodies
   c. IGM

4. Defects occur in 25% of offspring infected in first trimester

B. Cytomegalovirus

   1. Symptoms - usually none. May have mononucleosis-like syndrome

   2. Diagnosis - No practical way. Can be made by changes in indirect fluorescent antibody titer if known exposure has occurred. Virus can be cultured but are slow growing (weeks)

   3. Fetal effects
      a. Deafness or mental retardation occurs in 5-15% of congenitally infected infants.

   4. Significance
      a. CMV can be found in urine or cervix of 10-15% of mothers at term
      b. 40% of infants will develop neonatal infection - no known sequelae
      c. 4% of neonates will have + urine culture
      d. Estimates are that 1-2% of neonates have congenital infection

   5. Treatment - none known

C. Toxoplasmosis

   1. Symptoms
      a. May have lymphadenopathy
      b. Majority of infections are asymptomatic

   2. Diagnosis
      a. Lymph node biopsy
      b. Indirect fluorescent antibody (IgG and IGM)
      c. Sabin - Feldman dye test

   3. Incidence
      a. Chronic asymptomatic infection in 50% of population
      b. Only acute infection causes neonatal effects

   4. Fetal effects
      a. 98% end with normal offspring
      b. 2% show ocular or cerebellar lesions, stillbirth, or mental retardation

   5. Treatment
      a. Pyrimethamine and sulfadiazine in combination
      b. In two small series, treatment was begun antepartum, with no ill effects. However, teratogenicity of drugs is unknown and most authorities recommend treatment at birth if infant is infected.

ANTEPARTUM FETAL SURVEILLANCE

I. **Antepartum Fetal Heart Rate (FHR) Testing**

A. Purpose
1. To reduce the antepartum stillbirth rate
2. To screen for the presence of hypoxia and acidosis in the fetus

B. Indications
1. Postdates
2. Hypertension
3. Diabetes
4. Fetal growth abnormality
5. Rh isoimmunization
6. Amniotic fluid abnormality
7. Vaginal bleeding
8. Prior poor obstetric history

C. Types of tests
1. Nonstress test (NST)
   a. Definition: a pressure monitoring searching for adequate FHR accelerations during fetal movement
   b. Interpretation
      - Reactive: $\geq$ 2 accelerations (15 bpm above baseline for $\geq$ 15 sec. for 20 minutes)
      - Nonreactive: 0-1 adequate accelerations for 20 minutes
   c. Evaluation of nonreactive result: reassess underlying condition; repeat NST later in day, perform CST, or do biophysical profile (BPP)

2. Contraction Stress Test (CST)
   a. Definition: searching for late-onset FHR decelerations during uterine contractions
   b. Contraindications: Any contraindication to labor (ex: placenta previa, ruptured membranes); permissible if prior uterine surgery or active genital herpes
   c. Interpretation:
      - Negative: no late decelerations during 3 contractions over 10 min.
      - Suspicious: occasional late or variable decelerations during contraction
      - Positive: Late FHR decelerations coincident with contraction
   d. Evaluation of positive result: Reassess underlying condition and gestational age; repeat test later in day, perform biophysical profile or deliver

II.   Biophysical Profile Testing

Biophysical variable	Score	Explanation
Fetal breathing movements (FBM)	Normal = 2	≥1 FBM ≥30 sec duration in 30 minutes
	Abnormal = 0	No FBM ≥30 sec. duration in 30 minutes
Gross body movement	Normal = 2	≥3 discrete body/limb movements in 30 minutes
	Absent = 0	≥2 discrete body/limb movements in 30 minutes
Fetal tone	Normal = 2	≥1 episode active extension with return to flexion of fetal limbs/ trunk or opening/closing of hand
	Absent = 0	Either slow extension with return to partial flexion or movement of limb in full extension or absent feal movement
Reactive fetal heart rate	Normal = 2	Reactive NST
	Absent = 0	Nonreactive NST
Qualitative amniotic fluid volume	Normal = 2	≥1 pocket of amniotic fluid ≥1 cm in two perpendicular planes
	Absent = 0	No amniotic fluid or no pockets of fluid >1 cm in two perpendicular planes

A..   Interpretation of score
1.   0-4: consider delivery
2.   6: reassess, repeat test
3.   8-10: reassure

B..   Advantages
1.   Allows for more complete evaluation of fetus

III.   Amniotic Fluid Volume Assessment

A.   Methods
1.   Measure of single deep vertical pocket of fluid
2.   Measure of deepest vertical pocket of fluid in each of four quadrants of uterine cavity (amniotic fluid index - AFI)

B.   Definition of oligohydramnios
1.   AFI $\leq$ 5
2.   No amniotic fluid or no pockets >1 cm in two perpendicular planes

C.   Significance
1.   Uteroplacental insufficiency
2.   Fetal growth delay, pulmonary hypoplasia
3.   Umbilical cord compression

D.   Limitations
1.   Falsely abnormal result rates are often high (necessarily) to avoid falsely normal test results
2.   Underlying fetal or maternal condition may change leading to different results
3.   Often unable to predict acute event (placenta abruption, umbilical cord entanglement)

IV.   Obstetric Ultrasound

A.   Type of machines
1.   Real-time machines are used to visualize motion as well as anatomy
2.   Machines are portable to permit viewing in the clinic, ward, and labor and delivery areas

B.   Applications
1.   Confirm intrauterine pregnancy

2.   Basic (Level I) scan
    a.   Sac seen as early as 5th week using transvaginal transducer and 6th week using transabdominal transducer
    b.   Gestational age dating
    c.   Number of fetuses
    d.   Fetal presentation
    e.   Placental location
    f.   Amniotic fluid volume
    g.   Gross anomalies
        1)   Hydrocephaly
        2)   Anencephaly
        3)   Abdominal wall defect
    h.   Fetal viability
    i.   Fetal biometry
        1)   Biparietal diameter
        2)   Head circumference
        3)   Abdominal circumference
        4)   Femur length
    j.   Guidance for amniocentesis

      3.   Indications for the advanced (Level II) scan
         a.   Prior anomalous infant: rule out recurrence
         b.   Hydramnios: scan for anomalies
         c.   Oligohydramnios: scan for anomalies
         d.   Abnormal MSAFP
             1)   If high, rule out open neural tube defect or abdominal wall defect
             2)   If low, rule out chromosomally abnormal fetus
         e.   Abnormal growth
             1)   Small for gestation age: asymmetrical, symmetrical
             2)   Large for gestational age

    4.   Assessment of fetal well-being
         a.   Amniotic fluid volume
         b.   Biophysical profile testing

V.   Fetal Maturity Testing

    A.   When preterm delivery is a possibility

    B.   As adjunct to overall clinical assessment of maternal and fetal well-being and clinical gestational dating

    C.   Lung testing
        1.   Measure phospholipid levels which are important for surfactant synthesis (surface active material in lungs necessary to prevent alveolar collapse)
         a.   Lecithin/sphingomyelin
         b.   Phosphatidylglycerol

        2.   For predicting risk of respiratory distress syndrome (RDS)
         a.   Should be 2% or less if evidence of maturity
         b.   Only half of infants with an immature result will have RDS

    D.   Ultrasonic
        1.   Maturity strongly suggested if $\geq$ 39 weeks and biparietal diameter > 92 mm or grade III placenta

        2.   Estimated fetal weight as a sign of maturity is imprecise

VI.   Other

    A.   Fetal movement charting
        1.   A daily means of outpatient fetal assessment which enlists patient cooperation
        2.   Reassuring if less than one hour each day is necessary to count 10 movements
        3.   Requires FHR monitoring or a biophysical profile if fetus is perceived as being inactive
        4.   May be useful in both low and high risk pregnancy management

    B.   Fetal echocardiography

1.   Usually performed between 20-24 weeks
2.   To rule out complex heart defects
3.   Indications
        a.   Prior child with cardiac defect
        b.   Maternal diabetes
        c.   Maternal seizure disorder requiring medications.
        d.   Fetal arrhythmia evaluation

DIABETES AND PREGNANCY

I. Physiologic Changes During Pregnancy

A. Placental counterinsulin hormones (pregnancy is diabetogenic)
1. Human placental lactogen (HPL), estrogen, progesterone

B. Accelerated starvation of pregnancy
1. More prone to hypoglycemia if prolonged fasting (i.e. overnight fasting)

C. Effect on glucose tolerance curves
1. Slight changes during pregnancy: fasting level lower, one and two postprandial hour higher

II. Risks During Pregnancy

A. Maternal
1. Hypo and hyperglycemia, ketoacidosis
2. Infection-respiratory , urinary tract
3. Preeclampsia
4. Cesarean delivery

B. Fetal
1. Spontaneous abortion, stillbirth
2. Anomalies - especially cardiac and open neural tube defects
3. Large for gestational age; macrosomia near or at term

C. White classification
A_1 - Gestational onset, diet controlled
A_2 - Gestational onset, insulin requiring
B - Insulin dependent, < 10 years duration or > 20 year old at onset
C - Insulin dependent, 10-19 years duration or 10-19 year old at onset
D - Insulin dependent, 20 years duration or < 10 years old at onset
F - Insulin dependent with renal disease
R - Insulin dependent with proliferative retinopathy

III. Gestational Onset Diabetes Mellitus (GODM)

A. Screen
1. Risk factors
a. Family history, prior GODM, poor obstetric history, prior fetal macrosomia

2. 1-hr glucose challenge
a. Routinely perform on all patients at 24-28 weeks
b. Perform earlier and more often if other risk factors

        c.   Serum glucose > 140 mg% after 50-gm glucose load (15% of patients)require 3-hr glucose tolerance test

B.   Diagnosis: 3-hr oral glucose tolerance test
    1.   Definitive means to diagnose (2-3% of pregnant patients)
    2.   Requires $\geq$ 2 elevated serum glucose values (FBS, 1-,2-,&3-hour glucose samples)

C.   Patient profile
    1.   May be anyone
    2.   Often obese with high fat and refined carbohydrate diet

D.   Therapy
    1.   Diet
        a.   35 kcal/kg ideal body weight/day; usually 1800-2400 kcal/d
        b.   Calorie distribution: 50% carbohydrate (complex), 30% fat, 80-100 gm protein

    2.   Glucose monitoring
        a.   Usually fasting and 2-hour postprandial glucoses on semi-weekly basis in office or home (using reflectance dextrometer)
        b.   Would like values between 60-120

    3.   Insulin therapy
        a.   If diet alone is inadequate
        b.   Usual dose is eventually 0.5 U/kg/d in first trimester, 0.6 U/kg/d in 2nd trimester, 0.7 U/kg/d in third trimester
        c.   Divided into two or three doses each day using an intermediate acing (NPH or short acting (regular) insulin which is a recombinant DNA preparation (Humulin)

    4.   Fetal assessment
        a.   MSAFP at 15-20 weeks, fetal echocardiogram at 20-24 weeks
        b.   Periodic ultrasounds to estimate fetal weight and amniotic fluid volume
        c.   Daily fetal movement charting; weekly or semi-weekly nonstress tests in third trimester

    5.   Timing of delivery
        a.   Usually induction of labor by "due" date if uncomplicated
        b.   Once fetal lung maturity if chronic complications
        c.   Any time if acutely deteriorating maternal or fetal condition
        d.   Fetal macrosomia

IV.   Insulin Dependent Diabetes (IDDM)

A.   Management principles
    1.   Similar to gestational onset diabetic except preconception onset, more long-term problem, need for stricter control and more frequent monitoring

    B.   Initial evaluation/hospitalization
        1.   Baseline tests
            a.   Serum Hgb, A_1C, 24-hr urine for creatinine clearance and protein, retinal exam, EKG (if necessary)

        2.   Strict glucose control
            a.   Glucose levels < 100 mg% fasting and < 120 mg% at 2-hour postprandially

        3.   Patient education
            a.   More frequent glucose measurements and office visits
            b.   Improvements or refinements in diet
            c.   Earlier notification if any complications

    C.   Subsequent clinic visits
        1.   Glucose control (strict, fair, poor)
            a.   Always desired and sought upon reviewing daily diary

        2.   Anticipated insulin changes
            a.   Total daily dose is doubled or tripled during pregnancy in gradual manner

        3.   Fetal assessment
            a.   Same as GODM except nonstress testing may begin before 32 weeks and be more frequent

        4.   Timing of delivery
            a.   Same as GODM except usually induce labor once fetal lung maturity (usually > 37 weeks) unless strict glucose control

V.   Neonatal Concerns

    A.   Metabolic
        1.   Hypoglycemia, hypocalcemia, hyperbilirubinemia

    B.   Respiratory
        1.   Transient tachypnea, hyaline membrane disease

    C.   Anomalies
        1.   3-4 fold higher (from 2% → 8%)
        2.   Most often cardiac (septal defects. intraventricular hypertrophy) or open neural tube defects

    D.   Trauma
        1.   From failure to progress due to fetal size
        2.   Shoulder dystocia of particular concern if fetal macrosomia (≥4000 gm)
        3.   Midforceps delivery is discouraged

VI.   Future Childbearing

    A.   If already insulin dependent, recommend

          1.   Minimizing family size

          2.   Carefully planning pregnancies and discourage until
                a.   No other active medical disease(s)
                b.   Well controlled serum glucose levels

    B.   If gestational onset, recommend
          1.   Screening for diabetes at 6 week postpartum visit
          2.   Preconception counselling: screen for diabetes again, search for any other risk factors (obesity, hypertension, renal disease)

HYPERTENSION IN PREGNANCY

I. **Definition**

    A.   Hypertension
        1.   Diastolic pressure of 90 mm Hg or greater or systolic pressure of 140 mm Hg or greater, or a rise of diastolic pressure of at least 15 mm Hg or systolic pressure of at least 30 mm Hg

    B.   Chronic hypertension
        1.   Hypertension before 20 weeks gestation or beyond six weeks postpartum

    C.   Pregnancy-induced hypertension
        1.   Hypertension during second half of pregnancy without proteinuria or edema
        2.   Also known as transient, labile, or gestational hypertension

    D.   Preeclampsia
        1.   Hypertension with proteinuria or edema in second half of pregnancy
            a.   Mild preeclampsia: blood pressure less than 160/110 mmHg or 400 mg to 5 g protein /24 hr urine
            b.   Severe preeclampsia: blood pressure $\geq$ 160/110 mmHg or 5g protein/24 hr urine protein
            c.   Eclampsia: preeclampsia with seizure

II. **Incidence**

    A.   2-12% of pregnancies depending on population

    B.   Pregnancy onset more common than chronic hypertension

III. **Risks**

    A.   Maternal
        1.   Cerebrovascular accident, heart failure, hepatocellular dysfunction, renal failure, death

    B.   Fetal
        1.   Growth delay, hypoxia, intolerance to labor, death

IV. **Principles of Therapy**

    A.   Office visits
        1.   Maternal
            a.   Symptoms: visual disturbance, headache, right upper quadrant pain
            b.   Signs: elevated blood pressures using properly fitting blood pressure cuff; positioning (lateral reclining), and activity (rest) lowers readings; weight gain:

      c.   Watching for signs of superimposed preeclampsia: any of above with proteinuria

    2.   Laboratory tests

      a.   Maternal studies; complete blood count: increasing hematocrit; platelet count, coagulation profile (PT, PTT), fibrin split products:thrombocytopenia and coagulopathy

      b.   Liver function studies (hapatocellaelar dysfunction) and 24-h urine for creatine clearance and total urinary protein:(decreased renal function)

      c.   Fetal ultrasound for fetal weight and growth (small for gestational age), amniotic fluid volume (oligohydramnios), and placental status (accelerated calcification)

      d.   Fetal biophysical testing; NST/OCT, biophysical profile (inadequate oxygenation; acidosis, central nervous dysfunction)

B.   Drug therapy

    1.   Outpatient

      a.   Methyldopa (Aldomet) 250 mg b.i.d to 500 mg q.i.d.

      b.   Labetalol 100 mg b.i.d.

    2.   Magnesium sulfate

      a.   To avoid eclamptic seizures

      b.   4-g loading dose intravenously over 20-30 min. followed by 1-3 g/h

C.   When to admit

    1.   When expectant management at home does not result in normalization of blood pressure

    2.   Hospitalization offers better compliance in a more controlled environment

D.   Timing of delivery

    1.   When risk of permanent disability or death to the mother without intervention outweighs the risk to the fetus caused by intervention

      a.   Worsening of maternal condition

      b.   Fetal distress: when the intrauterine environment provides more risk to the fetus than delivery and care in the nursery

      c.   Fetal lung maturity

V. Recurrence Risk/Future Childbearing

A.   Chronic hypertension

    1.   Preconceptually - assess degree of blood pressure elevation and any end organ damage (renal, liver)

    2.   High if elevated blood pressures beyond 6 weeks postpartum, especially if requires medication

B.   Pregnancy induced

    1.   2-30% recurrence if mild preeclampsia; 15-30% recurrence if severe preeclampsia

    2.   Preconceptually search for any signs of hypertension or impaired renal function

Rh AND OTHER ISOIMMUNIZATION

I.   **Definition** - Isoimmunization is the development of antibodies to blood group antigens.

     A.   Serology

         1.   Major blood group isoantigens are proteins carried on the red cell membrane (A , B antigens). Because these antigens are very common in our environment (pollens, food, etc.), our immune system develops antibodies to these antigens - but only to those that are not present on the person's blood cell membranes.

         2.   These antibodies appear within a few months following birth. Type A persons have type A antigens on their red cells and have anti B (but not Anti A) antibodies in their serum. Similarly type B individuals have Anti A antibodies. Type O individuals (universal donors) have neither antigen on their red cells and develop both anti A and Anti B antibodies. The reverse is true for Type AB individuals (universal recipients) who carry neither antibody.

         3.   Rh Isoantigens - 85% of Caucasians (less common in Blacks or Orientals) have the Rh antigen on their red cell membranes. 15% do not have it and are termed Rh negative. The antigen is not found elsewhere in nature, so Rh negative individuals do not automatically develop antibodies to the Rh antigen (or "Factor") unless they are exposed to it by way of a blood transfusion with Rh positive blood, or, more commonly in women, exposed to small numbers of red blood cells from their fetus that cross the placenta into the mother's circulation, usually at birth.

     B.   Pathophysiology -

         1.   The "Rh Disease" results from the Rh negative mother becoming isoimmunized to an Rh antibody from the red cells of her first child.

             a.   The first Rh positive pregnancy is almost never affected unless the mother has had a previous blood transfusion with Rh positive blood.

             b.   Once immunized, the mother's immune system responds by manufacturing anti Rh isoantibodies with a second pregnancy.

             c.   If the second pregnancy is one in which the fetus is Rh positive, the mother's anti Rh Isoantibodies are transferred to the fetus across the placenta.

         2.   Once in the fetal blood, the Rh isoantibodies react with the Rh antigen on the fetal red cell, marking it for destruction by the fetal spleen.

             a.   There is a general relationship between the number of antibodies produced by the mother ("her anti Rh titer") and the number of fetal red cells destroyed.

             b.   Thus an Rh negative mother sensitized to the Rh antigen by a previous pregnancy may have mounted a very strong immune response, and produced a large number of anti Rh antibodies. In such a case, an anti Rh antibody titer ("Coomb's titer") will be "high"; the number of antibody molecules that cross the placenta will be high and the fetus will have many red cells destroyed.

    c.   In many cases with a high anti Rh titer, the fetal bone marrow response to the red cell destruction will not be adequate to prevent the development of fetal anemia.

3.   If the fetal anemia is severe enough, the fetus will go into heart failure and develop "hydrops fetalis". Hydropic fetuses usually die in utero or soon after birth.

4.   If the Rh positive fetus of an Rh isoimmunized mother is born alive and not in heart failure, one of several clinical pictures may be produced:

    a.   Anemia: may be severe or not severe enough to require treatment.

    b.   Jaundice: Because of the fetal blood destruction, the newborn will usually develop jaundice. Jaundice occurs because the increased red cell destruction releases larger amounts of hemoglobin than normal. Hemoglobin is broken down to bilirubin pigments, which normally would be metabolized by the liver to form bilirubin glucuronide. In the fetus the excess bilirubin is passed back through the placenta and the mother's liver excretes it into her bile. In the newborn, the glucuronase transferase enzyme system in the liver is not mature enough to metabolize the larger amounts of bilirubin. Bilirubin thus builds up in the blood, producing the typical bronzed color of the skin we recognize as "jaundice"

    c.   Kernicterus (brain damage caused by bilirubin): Most bilirubin is bound to albumin in the newborn's blood. When the concentration of bilirubin in the newborn's blood exceeds 20 mg %, the albumin binding sites are all filled, and bilirubin molecules are then freed to enter the tissues. Bilirubin is a cytologic poison, and it is preferentially taken up by the cells of the basal ganglia. When a sufficient number of basal ganglia neurons are damaged by the larger amount bilirubin, the function of the basal ganglia is destroyed. The clinical picture is one of motor handicap (similar to cerebral palsy). Once this pathophysiology was understood, methods of management and later prevention were developed.

II.   Management

    A.   During pregnancy:

        1.   Establish Rh status of all pregnant women at first prenatal visit.

        2.   If the woman is Rh negative, find out if her husband or the father of this pregnancy is Rh positive or negative. If unsure, treat patient as if the father of the fetus is Rh positive.

        3.   If the mother is Rh negative test to see if she has anti Rh isoantibodies (the "indirect Coomb's test" or "antibody screening test").

        4.   If no antibodies found - see prevention.

5.   If mother has Rh Isoantibodies, perform titer to see if she has mild or severe Isoimmunization.

a.   Mild Isoimmunization - antibody titer below 1:16 in most laboratories. Titers this low rarely produce fetal hydrops and usually do not require any intervention in the pregnancy. The newborn however, may be anemic and develop hyperbilirubinemia.

b.   Severe isoimmunization: Titers of over 1:16 may produce significant anemia in utero, and those over 1:256 may produce hydrops. Severe isoimmunization requires an estimate of how severe the fetal anemia is. This should be done in the 2nd trimester, and may consist of an amniocenteses or percutaneous umbilical blood sampling (PUBS).

c.   Amniocentesis denotes the amount of blood destruction by estimating the amount of bilirubin pigments in the fluid. Using the "Liley" method, there is a surprisingly good correlation between the "450 mu peak" and the amount of fetal anemia

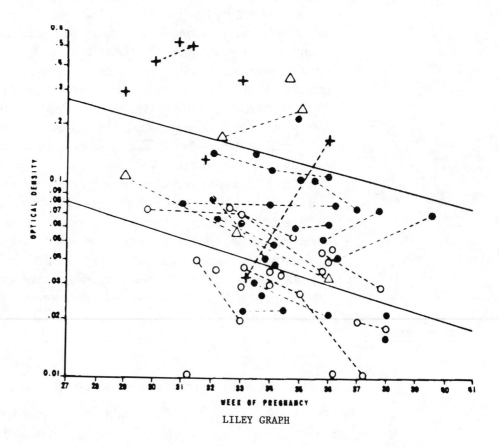

LILEY GRAPH

6.   Fetuses in the low zone rarely are sick if born at term. Those in the lower mid zone are sometimes symptomatic if born at term. To determine the best time for delivery, they are usually followed by repeated amniocentesis. In the upper mid zone, weekly amniocentesis may allow the pregnancy to be followed until the amount of bilirubin seen enters the upper zone. Most fetuses in the upper zone

will die within a week or 10 days, and should be delivered in a tertiary care center promptly.

7. Occasionally a fetus is found in the upper zone, but is so early in gestation (24 to 28 weeks) that prompt delivery would by itself have a high mortality. In such cases intrauterine blood transfusions are done.

B. Following Birth: After birth, the hemoglobin level in the newborn may be so low as to require blood transfusions. Sometimes the newborn is so anemic, an immediate transfusion my be life saving. To be properly prepared for this emergency, during labor type O negative blood is cross matched against the mother (it is she from whom all of the fetus's Isoantibodies come). When there is no emergency, the blood may be Rh negative but of the newborn's major blood group type.

The bilirubin level in newborn's blood is usually measured frequently in the first few days after birth. If the level exceeds certain critical levels the newborn may need an exchange transfusion in which blood is removed and bank blood transfused. This process removes bilirubin and isoantibodies and corrects the anemia. Exchange transfusions are very well tolerated by newborns.

III. Prevention.

A. It has been shown that Rh positive cells will not produce an immune response in an Rh negative woman if the anti Rh isoantibodies (RhoGAM) are injected into the mother within 72 hours. Thus if anti Rh isoantibodies can be injected into Rh negative woman carrying an Rh positive fetus within 72 hours of birth, the initial sensitization of the Rh negative mother to the Rh positive fetal cells can be prevented. This technique 98-99% effective in preventing Rh isoimmunization. To further increase the effectiveness, a similar dose (300mg) of Rh immune globulin is also administered at the end of the second trimester. With both injections, less than 1% of Rh negative women carrying Rh positive fetuses become Rh isoimmunized today.

PREMATURE LABOR
PRETERM RUPTURE OF MEMBRANES

I. **Definitions**

    A.   Premature: 20-37 weeks 6 days

    B.   Premature rupture of membranes: ruptured membranes before labor

    C.   Preterm rupture of membranes: ruptured membranes before 37 completed weeks

    D.   Premature labor: regular uterine contractions between 20 and 37 weeks gestation

    E.   Low birth weight: 2500 g or less

    F.   Very low birth weight: 1500 g or less

II. **Incidence**

    A.   10% and accounts for 50-70% of perinatal morbidity and mortality

    B.   Has not changed in last 40 years despite multiple therapy attempts

III. **Etiology/Initial Evaluation**

	Conditions	Tests
Maternal	• active medical disorder • dehydration • infection (urinary,cervical) • substance abuse	• complete blood count • history,physical • urine & cervical/vaginal cultures (n. gonorrhea, chlamydia, group B streptococcus) • urine drug screen
Uteroplacental	• placenta previa, abruption • ruptured membranes • incompetent cervix • hydramnios • uterine distortion (fibroids,septum) • intra-amniotic infection	• ultrasound • pelvic exam • amniocentesis
Fetal	• major anomalies • twins	• ultrasound • amniocentesis

IV. Diagnosis

    A. Preterm rupture of membranes
        1. History of "gush" of fluid
        2. "Pooling" of fluid intravaginally
        3. Laboratory evidence: nitrazine positive, "ferning" or sodium crystal formation

    B. Premature labor
        1. Regular uterine contractions lasting at least 30 seconds with a frequency of 1 in every 10 minutes of less
        2. Does not require cervical dilation(unlike labor at term)

    C. Observation
        1. Over 50% of premature labor will resolve with hydration and bedrest

V. Therapeutic Considerations

    A. Gestational age
        1. Consider no treatment if before "viability" (< 24 weeks) or beyond 33 weeks
        2. Tocolysis and possible antibiotics if 24-33 weeks

    B. Fetal lung maturity
        1. Tocolysis if results of amniotic fluid testing of phospholipid levels (L/S, PG) are immature

    C. Evidence for infection
        1. No tocolysis in presence of fetal tachycardia; maternal fever, uterine tenderness, persistent labor
        2. Begin broad spectrum antibiotics and induce labor if diagnosis is reasonably certain

    D. Other underlying conditions
        1. Maternal: poorly controlled diabetes, severe preeclampsia
        2. Fetal: active vaginal bleeding, abnormal heart rate pattern, lethal anomaly

VI. Drug Therapy

    A. Tocolytic therapy
        1. Types
        2. Contraindication
            a. Active vaginal bleeding, abnormal fetal heart rate pattern, active medical disorder, advanced labor, lethal fetal anomalies

Class and action	Comments
Magnesium sulfate Competes with calcium for entry into cells	High degree of safety. Often used as first agent. May cause flushing or headaches. At high levels may cause respiratory depression (12-15 mg/dl) or cardiac depression (> 15 mg/dl).
β *-Adrenergic agents* (ritodrine, terbutaline) Increases cyclic AMP in cell, which decreases free calcium	β-Receptors are of two types: β_1 predominate in heart intestines; β_2 predominate in the uterus, lungs, and blood vessels. Side effects include hypotension, tachycardia, anxiety, chest tightening or pain, ECG changes; also increased pulmonary edema very in-frequently but possible, especially with fluid overload.
Prostaglandin synthetase inhibitors (indomethacin) Decrease prostaglandin (PG) production by blocking conversion of free arachidonic acid to PG	Premature constriction of ductus arteriosus possible especially after 34 weeks; bradycardia, growth re- tardation hypoglycemia reported earlier, but concern has decreased with broader experience.
Calcium channel blockers (nifedipine) Prevent calcium entry into muscle cells	Newest tocolytic; possible decrease in uteroplacental blood flow, fetal hypoxia, hypercarbia. More ex perience needed.

        3.   Discontinue when any undesired side effects, evidence of lung maturity, persistent contractions

B.   Antibiotics
        1.   May aid when infection suspected
        2.   To reduce infant infection
        3.   Ampicillin and gentamicin

C.   Corticosteroids
        1.   Between 26 and 32 weeks
        2.   To enhance fetal lung maturity
        3.   Betamethasone 12 mg for 2 doses (12-24 hr. apart)

VII. Recurrence Risk

A.   Later in gestation
        1.   Higher if noncorrectible cause or idiopathic labor
        2.   Greater than if no premature labor before

B.   Subsequent pregnancies
        1.   Greater when cause of premature labor is unknown or apt to recur
        2.   15% if occurred with one prior pregnancy, 25% if two prior pregnancies

THIRD TRIMESTER BLEEDING

I. Background

A. Definition: any vaginal bleeding late in pregnancy

B. Greatest concerns involve a placental abnormality
   1. Placental abruption: separation of the placenta from the uterine wall
   2. Placenta previa: low lying placenta which is covering the internal cervical os

II. Differential Diagnosis

	Maternal Signs & Symptoms	Ultrasonic Findings
Placental abruption Central Marginal	Cramping; contractions Bleeding alone	May be nonspecific; increased thickness of placenta Usually low-lying placenta
Placenta previa Complete/total Marginal	Intermittent bleeding; may become profuse Intermittent bleeding	Placenta totally covering internal cervical os Placental edge at or very close to internal cervical os
Early labor	Accompanying contractions; bloody mucus discharge	Nonspecific
Coagulopathy	Prolonged time to form any clot	Nonspecific
Gynecologic cervical polyp, cancer; hemorrhoids; cervicitis	Spotting: may be postcoital or after bowel movement	Nonspecific

III. Hazards

A. Maternal
   1. Mild: anemia, fatigue, transfusion
   2. Severe: shock, death, transfusion

B. Fetal
   1. Mild: growth delay
   2. Severe: hypoxia, demise, growth delay

IV. Initial Evaluation

A. Ultrasound evaluation

B. Pelvic exam: external and speculum inspection

C.   Continuous fetal heart rate and uterine activity monitoring

D.   Coagulation studies: PTT, PIT, fibrinogen, platelet count

V.   Therapy (General Principles)

A.   Placental abruption
1.   Expectant management
     a.   Observe for worsening of any underlying condition
     b.   Monitor for abnormal fetal heart rate pattern (bradycardia, later decelerations), and labor
2.   Allow for vaginal delivery if adequate progress and tolerated by fetus

B.   Placenta previa
1.   Transfuse to hemoglobin 10 mg %
2.   Deliver by cesarean section if profuse vaginal blooding or fetal lung maturity at or near term

VI.   Management of Shock

A.   Monitor closely: vital signs, urine output, fetal heart rate

B.   Elevate foot of table or bed

C.   Plasma expanders such as Lactated ringers' or normal saline are used.

D.   A minimum of 1 unit of packed red blood cells or whole blood should be transfused

E.   Transfuse with platelets (6-10 packs to increase count 15-60,000/mm^2), cryoprecipitate, or fresh frozen plasma (usually 4 units)

MULTIFETAL GESTATION

I. Incidence

    A. One in 90 pregnancies
        1. Monozygotic 1 in 250

    B. Only half detected in first trimester survive as twins

II. Mechanics of Twinning

    A. Monozygotic (identical) division of fertilized ovum

    B. Dizygotic (fraternal)
        1. Two separate ova fertilized by two sperm
        2. Increasing maternal age, increasing parity, family history (maternal)
        3. Fertility drugs: clomiphene 6-8%, exogenous gonadotropins 15-25%
        4. In vitro fertilization 35-40%

III. Overview of Risk Factors

	Antepartum	Intrapartum	Postpartum
Maternal	Accelerated physiologic changes Hypertension Diabetes Anemia	Cesarean section Hemorrhage Prolonged labor Premature labor	Infection Anemia Breast feeding limitations Delayed recovery Adjustment difficulties
Fetal/Neonatal	Abortion Congenital anomalies Stillbirth Delayed or discordant growth Twin-twin transfusion	Malpresentation Cord accident Intolerance to labor Trauma	Prematurity Low Apgars Trauma

IV. Antepartum Evaluation

    A. Clinic visits/examination
        1. Weekly, every other week
        2. Observe for above risk factors
        3. Periodic ultrasonography
        4. Nutrition, bedrest

B.   Laboratory tests
   1.   Routine
      a.   Complete blood count
      b.   Diabetes screen
      c.   Urinalysis, culture

   2.   Value of ultrasonography
      a.   Early diagnosis
      b.   Monoamniotic vs. diamniotic
      c.   Conjoined twins and other anomalies
      d.   Twin-twin transfusion, "stuck twin"
      e.   Growth assessment: each fetus and discordant ($\geq 20\%$ difference)
      f.   Biophysical assessment
      g.   Fetal presentations
      h.   Delivery of second twin (localizing heart rate, presentation)

V.   Delivery Considerations

A.   When
   1.   Worsening of any risk factors
   2.   Spontaneous labor at or near term
   3.   Progressing premature labor

B.   Route
   1.   More often by cesarean section
   2.   Consider vaginal delivery if cephalic/cephalic presentation
      a.   Unless very premature(?)
      b.   Second twin may still require cesarean delivery

VI.   Subsequent Pregnancies

A.   Recurrence risk very unlikely (1-2%)

B.   Risks with fertility drugs same

VII.   Triplet Pregnancy

A.   Approximately 1/8,100 pregnancies ($1/90^2$)

B.   Same risks as for twins but more often

C.   Delivery averages at 32 weeks (36 weeks for twins)

POSTTERM PREGNANCY

I. Scope of the Problem

A. Gestational dating
1. Between 2 and 11% of all pregnancies remain undelivered for 2 weeks or more beyond the due date
2. Approximately 40% have inaccurate dates

B. Perinatal morbidity
1. Immediate problems in the newborn: asphyxia, meconium aspiration, seizure disorders, metabolic imbalances, and respiratory difficulties
2. Between 12 and 43% (approximately 20% of patients with postterm pregnancies deliver infants with classic finding of dysmaturity or postmaturity
   a. These infants have long lean bodies with characteristic skin changes (leather-like consistency, little subcutaneous fat, and desquamation of the skin)
   b. Long hair, meconium staining, longer fingernails, and an alert facial expression may also be seen
   c. Although these infants are often heavier than average for a term pregnancy, these physical findings suggest a form of intrauterine growth retardation

II. Antepartum Management

A. Pregnancy dating
1. Last menstrual period, quickening, auscultation of fetal heart tones, serial uterine fundal height examination, and any ultrasound examination(s)
   a. With accurate gestational dating and the pregnancy now 2 weeks beyond the estimated date of confinement, a search for other complications and an examination of the cervix are indicated
2. If accurate dating is not possible or the cervix is "unripe", manage conservatively with semiweekly clinical visits and fetal biophysical   assessments.
3. Half will be expected to go into labor and delivery by 42 3/7 weeks, while 90% will deliver by 43 weeks

B. Fetal assessment
1. Fetal movement charting
   a. "Count to 10" method is easy to comprehend and use
2. Antepartum fetal heart rate testing
   a. A reactive nonstress test (2 or more adequate accelerations of the baseline fetal heart rate during a 20-40 minute period) should be repeated within the next week.
   b. A nonreactive result should be repeated that same day, or a contraction stress test should be performed.

    c.   The absence of fetal heart rate decelerations coincident with uterine activity is reassuring; when decelerations are detected, they suggest fetal compromise from cord compression or uteroplacental insufficiency

3.   Ultrasonography
    a.   Scan for the presence of any fetal malformations (anencephaly), gross fetal body movements, fetal respiratory movements, and amniotic fluid volume
    b.   Oligohydramnios is a warning sign of an increased risk of meconium, fetal acidosis, perinatal morbidity and mortality, and birth asphyxia
    c.   Amniotic fluid may be characterized as being adequate, pockets, or oligohydramnios (vertical pockets that are 2 cm deep or less, or a 4-quadrant amniotic fluid index < 5)

III.   Intrapartum Management

A.   If the cervix is ripe or there are any abnormal findings on clinical examination of fetal testing, delivery with optimal fetal monitoring is recommended.

B.   Once easily palpable, the amniotic membranes should be ruptured to permit internal monitoring of the fetal heart rate and uterine activity.

C.   Meconium is present in 25-30% of cases (compared to 10-15% at term) and is often thick.

D.   Any evidence of fetal distress (usually umbilical cord compression) requires observation, fetal acoustic stimulation, fetal scalp stimulation or scalp blood sampling, or prompt delivery

E.   Fetal heart rate patterns most suggestive of fetal compromise include: severe bradycardia, repetitive late decelerations, undulating baseline between tachycardia and bradycardia, and unexplained poor or absent beta-to-beat variability

F.   Internal uterine pressure catheters permit the amnioinfusion of 1,000 ml or more of normal saline in the presence of meconium, variable deceleration, or oligohydramnios.

G.   Approximately 25% of postdate pregnancies will have a macrosomic (> 4000 g) fetus.
1.   Between 2.5 and 10% of postdate pregnancies will carry a fetus weighing 4500 g or more.

H.   There is an approximate 20% chance of primary cesarean section or need for forceps delivery

FETAL DEATH

I. Definitions

    A. Abortion
        1. Loss of pregnancy before 20 weeks gestation or weight < 500 gm

    B. Fetal death
        1. Lack of fetal heart rate at or beyond 20 weeks gestation
        2. Approximately 9/1,000 births
        3. Usually antepartum not intrapartum

    C. Neonatal death
        1. Occurs from birth up to 28 days

    D. Perinatal death
        1. Fetal plus neonatal deaths
            a. Rate reported per 1000 total births
            b. Neonatal death - infant death in first 7 days, expressed as rate per 1,000 live births; usually similar rate or slightly less than fetal death

    E. Maternal mortality
        1. 10 per 100,000 live births
        2. Cause is either directly from obstetric disease (hypertension, hemorrhage), indirect if disease co-existing with pregnancy (renal failure) or nonmaternal(trauma, drug overdose)
        3. Up to 42 days (6 weeks) postpartum

II. Diagnosis

    A. Chief complaint - fetal movement not felt

    B. Lack of cardiac activity by auscultation
        1. Confirmed by real-time ultrasound with certainty by 8 weeks
        2. By Doppler at 10-12 weeks, by fetoscope at 18-20 weeks

    C. X-ray findings (overlapping skull bones, marked curvature of spine, gas in circulation):
        1. Unreliable
        2. Requires days to develop

III. Etiology

    A. Maternal
        1. Hypertension
        2. Diabetes
        3. Sepsis

B.   Uteroplacental
  1.   Abruption
  2.   Umbilical cord complication (entanglement, prolapse, etc.)

C.   Fetal
  1.   Infection: TORCH, Listeria, group B streptococcus
  2.   Chromosome: monosomy, trisomy, polyploidy
  3.   Multifetal gestation

D.   Unknown
  1.   Particularly true late in gestation

IV.   Complications

A.   Emotional ramifications
  1.   Usually desire shortly time after diagnosis

  2.   Grief response: hostility, denial, eventual acceptance

  3.   Counseling
    a.   Should overcome loss
    b.   Crying, sleeping problems, eating difficulties usually temporary
    c.   Consider spouse's welfare also

B.   Morbidity
  1.   Infection from retained products
    a.   Uncommon
    b.   Antibiotics and uterine evaluation

  2.   Coagulopathy
    a.   Retained tissue beyond 4 weeks
    b.   From thromboplastin release into maternal circulation
        1.   Leads to hypofibrinogenemia
    c.   Weekly serum fibrinogen and fibrin degration products

V.   Uterine Evacuation

A.   Gestational age
  1.   < 20 weeks (missed abortion): dilation and evacuation vs. 20-mg prostaglandin E2 vaginal suppositories

  2.   20-27 weeks: prostaglandin E2 vaginal suppositories

  3.   ≥ 28 weeks: prostaglandin E2 gel to ripen cervix and oxytocin infusion

B.   No role for hysterectomy or hysterotomy unless preexisting gynecologic disease or rapidly deteriorating maternal illness

VI. Examination of Stillbirth and Placenta

A. Rule out abruption, cord entanglement, 2 cord vessels, abnormal cord insertion

B. Search for external fetal anomalies (face, spine, external genitalia, imperforate anus, extremities

C. Consent for an autopsy - renal, hepatic, cardiac

D. Request a placental microscopic examination - chronic inflammation, vascular changes

E. Obtain cells for fetal karyotyping - amniotic fluid, fetal blood, skin, amnion

POSTPARTUM HEMORRHAGE

I.   **Definition**

   A.   More than 500 mL after a vaginal delivery or 800 mL during a cesarean section

   B.   Diagnosed by clinical suspicion

II.   **Causes and Their Predisposing Factors:**

   A   Uterine
   1.   Atony - over distended uterus, rapid labor, infection
   2.   Retained placental fragments - prematurity, manual removal of placenta
   3.   Tear - prior uterine surgery, uterine hyperstimulation

   B.   Lacerations (cervix, vagina, perineum) - large fetus, rapid delivery, operative delivery, forceps or vacuum

   C.   Coagulopathy - inherited, drug-induced, toxemia, fetal demise

   D.   Concealed pelvic hematoma - traumatic delivery

III.   **Management**

   A.   At or shortly after delivery
   1.   Conservative
      a.   Uterine massage
      b.   Inspection of placenta and lower genital tract
      c.   Inspection for clot formation
      d.   Coagulation studies

   2.   Uterine contracting drugs
      a.   Oxytocin (Pitocin) 10-20 units in intravenous solution
      b.   Methylergonovine (Methergine) - intramuscularly
      c.   Prostaglandin F2 alpha (Hemabate)-intramuscularly or intravenously

   3.   Surgery
      a.   Uterine curettage
      b.   Uterine artery/broad ligament compression
      c.   Hypogastric artery ligation
      d.   Hysterectomy

   B.   Delayed hemorrhage
   1.   Usually first two weeks postpartum
   2.   Causes: uterine atony, retained placental fragment
   3.   Treatment: oral methylergonovine vs. curettage

IV. **Recurrence Risk**

    A.   Consider etiology and any predisposing factors

    B.   Low chance of recurrence but higher than if no prior episode

    C.   Be prepared: adequate lighting, assistant, anesthesia available

POSTPARTUM FEVER

I. Definition

A. Temperature of 38° C (100.4°F) or higher on two occasions beyond the first 24 hours and within the next 9 days postpartum

II. Incidence

A. Variable: 2%-50%
 1. Lowest after a spontaneous vaginal delivery without prolonged ruptured membranes
 2. Highest after a cesarean section after prolonged ruptured membranes

III. Predisposing Factors

A. Rupture of fetal membranes

B. Intraamniotic infection

C. Prolonged labor

D. Multiple pelvic examinations

E. Obesity

F. Anemia

G. Prolonged operating time

H. Low socioeconomic status

IV. Differential diagnosis

Causes	Days after delivery	Primary signs or symptoms	Labs	Therapy
Wind Atelectasis	1st 24 h	Dyspnea	Chest x-ray	Respiratory therapy; antibiotics
Pneumonia	2-5 d			
Womb Endomyometritis	1-4 d	Uterine tenderness	Uterine cavity culture (limited value)	Broad spectrum single or combination antibiotics (cefotetan, cefoxitin, clindamycin and gentamicin)
Water Urinary tract infection	2-5 d	Dysuria, urinary frequency, costovertebral tenderness	Urine culture	Antibiotic;hydration
Wound Wound infection	3-7 d	Tenderness, fluctuation erythema	Wound culture	Open and drain; antibiotics against staph aureus
Wonder drug (usually antibiotic)	5-10 d	None	None	Discontinue drug
Walk Septic thrombophlebitis	3-7 d	Thigh tenderness; tachycardia	Impedance plesthesmography; CT scanning (if pelvic mass suspected)	Heparin; antibiotics
Women's breasts Noninfectious mastitis	≥ 7 d	tender, no discolor; symmetric; engorged breasts	None	Lactation suppressant; nonstimulation (tight bra, cold compresses)
Infectious Bacterial mastitis	≥ 14 d	Unilateral; tenderness; erythema	None	Antibiotic which is penicillinase-resistant

POSTPARTUM DEPRESSION

I.   **Postpartum "Blues" - up to 70%**

    A.   Occurs during first 2 weeks after delivery - usually 48-72 hours postpartum

    B.   Manifested by tearfulness, anxiety, mood lability, irritability, insomnia, depression.

    C.   No treatment required.

II.   **Postpartum Depression - Up to 15%**

    A.   Not related to social class, marital status, or parity.

    B.   Usually occurs in women with previous depressive diagnosis or other life situations predisposing them to depression.

    C.   Greater than 50% recurrence rate.

    D.   Shows symptoms of depression but also poor relationship with family and ambivalence toward the infant.

    E.   Initial treatment with tricyclic antidepressant (ex. Imiprimine)

    F.   Counseling of the family also important.

III.   **Postpartum Psychosis - <0.3%**

    A.   Usually lasts 2-3 months

    B.   Most show symptoms of manic - depressive type, with confusion and disorientation; delusional thoughts or expressions of suicide differentiate this from blues or depression.

    C.   Initial evaluation should be as an inpatient.

    D.   Medical therapy overall not extremely helpful. Most commonly used are tricyclic antidepressants, neuroleptics, lithium carbonate and electroconvulsive therapy.

GYNECOLOGY

HUMAN SEXUALITY

I. **Introduction**

    1.   Sexual dysfunctions are common problems

    2.   About one couple in five suffers from sexual dysfunction

    3.   Most common presentation is to a gynecologist

II. **Approach to the Patient**

    1.   Medical model

        a.   In a medical model, we traditionally look at an alteration of normal physiology leading to a disease state. We endeavor to find the cause of the pathophysiology and alter or remove the cause. The approach consists of history, physical examination, laboratory evaluation, diagnosis and therapy. Each physician decides what problems to evaluate or refer based on experience and ability.

        b.   Sexual problems can be addressed in a traditional medical model.

    2.   Application of medical model to sexual dysfunction

        a.   Normal sexual physiology

            1.   Sexual response is a natural physiologic response. It cannot be learned or taught, just as digestion, respiration, etc... cannot be learned or taught.

            2.   Phases of sexual response

    A.   Desire

        1.   Desire for intercourse is a primary desire like that for food, water or air

        2.   Some degree of desire is always present

        3.   Like all appetites, desire can be whetted or inhibited by circumstances

        4.   Sexual desire is not lust

    B.   Excitement

        1.   Vasocongestion

        2.   Shift in blood flow to pelvis

        3.   Increase in heart rate and respiration

        4.   Skin "mottling" and feeling of warmth

        5.   Nipple erection

        6.   Male - Penile erection, scrotal shortening

        7.   Female - Vaginal lubrication, expansion, clitoral vasocongestion

    C.   Plateau

        1.   Essentially a more advanced stage of arousal

        2.   Physiology remains unchanged for some time

        3.   No further increase in heart rate, respiration, blood flow shifts.

D. Orgasm
    1. Rhythmic contractions of perineal muscles (0.8 seconds)
    2. Male - Accompanied by 3 to 7 ejaculatory spurts
    3. Female - Accompanied by elevation of "orgasmic platform" contractions, EEG changes

E. Resolution
    1. Males:
        Orgasm is followed by an obligatory resolution phase in which physiologic changes return to baseline and further stimulation cannot produce excitement. Length varies with age - from < 5 minutes in adolescence to 24 hours or longer in elderly.

    2. Females:
        Resolution is not obligatory- women may have repeated orgasm without resolution to basal state, but some women do have obligatory resolution phase.

III. Sexual Dysfunctions

A. Manifested by alteration in normal physiologic response

B. May be due to psychological, physical or pharmacological factors.

C. Have anxiety as an essential component

D. Abnormal sexual physiology
    1. Result from "blocks" in normal physiology
    2. "Blocks" can be pain, spectating, "what's wrong with me?"

E. Desire phase
    1. Inhibited sexual desire
        a. ISD vs lack of desire. Many patients complain that they have no desire for intercourse. Careful history reveals that most of these have an inhibited desire for intercourse. Most will admit to a desire, but that in a sexual situation, they have an averse reaction. The most common etiology is pain - physical or psychic.
        b. ISD. Inhibited desire is a learned behavior - a conditioned response. It may be secondary to another dysfunction, pain, boredom, or anger/marital discord.

F. Excitement phase
    1. Erectile dysfunctions are manifested by failure of penile engorgement. They may be a result of vascular disease or performance anxiety.
    2. Premature ejaculation is a failure of excitement. Most men with premature ejaculation believe that they are too excited and try to limit excitement, which has the effect of making the problem worse.

3. Vaginismus is an involuntary spasm of the muscles around the lower third of the vagina. It may make penetration impossible. Vaginismus may be universal or situational and may be primary or secondary. The etiology is pain - either physical or psychological, Severe negative parenting about sexuality is often found.

4. Dyspareunia is pain with intercourse.
Dyspareunia may be due to physical causes - vaginitis, endometriosis, chronic pelvic inflammatory disease. It may be due to failure of excitement with failure of lubrication and vaginal expansion.

G. Plateau phase
1. Orgasmic dysfunction may be defined as inability to achieve orgasm. It may be situational or constant, primary or secondary. The etiology is usually performance anxiety although it may be due to inadequate clitoral stimulation or boredom or fear of loss of control.

2. Delayed ejaculation is the male equivalent of anorgasmia. It is usually due to performance anxiety.

H. Orgasm
1. Pain with orgasm is a rare condition that may be due to pelvic adhesions or tears in the endopelvic fascia.

I. Resolution
1. Prolonged resolution phases may lead to a false diagnosis of erectile dysfunction. In elderly men, the resolution phase may be prolonged enough to interfere with erection at a subsequent sexual encounter.

IV. Diagnosis

A. History
1. "What happens" ?
2. When?
3. Sexual ROS
   a. How often do you have intercourse?
   b. Do you have pain with intercourse
   c. How often do you have orgasms with intercourse? (females)
   d. Do you ever have orgasm before you want to? (males)
   e. Do you ever have trouble getting or keeping an erection? (males)
   f. Are you generally satisfied with your sex life?

B. Physical examination
1. General physical
2. Pelvic examination

C. Determination of "internal theory"

1.   All patients have an internal theory of the cause and often treatment of their problem. Everything we tell them is filtered through this theory. We must discover this internal theory and if it is correct (we agree with it!) then fine. If not, we must educate the patient about our theory or at least persuade the patient to try our theory and therapy.

V. Therapy

A.   PLISSIT model
    1.   Permission giving
        a.   Many sexual problems can be managed with permission and education.
        b.   Examples - "It is OK to touch your clitoris during intercourse".
    2.   Limited Information
        a.   Education can resolve many problems.
        b.   Examples - "It is normal to have an erection every 90 minutes at night." "You don't have to be 'in the mood' to have intercourse"
    3.   Specific suggestions
        a.   Some problems may respond to specific suggestions
        b.   Examples - Try a lubricant. Try touching your clitoris. Tell your husband what you like or don't like.
    4.   Intensive therapy
        a.   Many dysfunctions will only respond to intensive therapy.
        b.   Traditional sex therapy - 12 - 16 visits, sensate focus.

B.   Every physician must decide what problems to manage and what to refer. As always, accurate diagnosis is the key to successful therapy.

CONTRACEPTION

I. Background

A.   Most Common Methods in U.S   #1   Sterilization
                                                    #2   Oral Contraceptives
                                                    #3   Condoms

B.   Contraception: Preventing pregnancy

C.   Effectiveness:
1.   Method effectiveness - when always used correctly
2.   Use effectiveness - rate in actual use for a specific method
3.   Effectiveness rate is the percentage of women using a method who do not conceive in one year

II. Methods

A.   Barrier

Type:	Condoms	Diaphragm	Sponge	Female Condom	Cervical Cap
Description Name	Sheath of latex or animal tissue that covers the penis to collect the semen	Dome-shaped rubber disc in various sizes	Today Sponge, disc-shaped sponge containing nonoxynol-9	Vaginal pouch, polyurethane sheath to cover female reproductive tract	Rubber cap
Mechanism of Action:	Forms a barrier that prevents sperm from entering the female reproductive tract	Covers cervix to block sperm entry into upper female reproductive trace, used with a spermicide	Placed in vagina over cervix as a barrier to sperm entering the female reproductive tract and kills them with spermicide	A barrier that prevents sperm entry into female reproductive tract	Covers cervix to block sperm entry into female reproductive tract, used with a spermicide
Advantage:	Over-the-counter, protect against STD's, inexpensive	Non-hormonal, STD protection, reusable, decreased dysplasia	Over-the-counter, can be placed hours before intercourse, some STD protection, effective up to 24 hours	Over-the counter, STD protection, more variety of placement time, no latex allergy	Non-hormonal, STD protection, reusable

A.   Barrier (cont.)

Type:	Condoms	Diaphragm	Sponge	Female Condom	Cervical Cap
Disadvantage (Side Effects)	Allergic reaction, decreased male sensation	May need to interrupt sexual activity to place, may dislodge during sex, allergy to rubber, inability to insert/remove, increased risk of bladder infections, requires fitting by health care professional, remain in place 6-8 hours	Allergic reaction, dislodge during sex, infection risk if not removed in 24 hours such as toxic shock syndrome	Insertion difficulty, dislodge during sex, vaginal irritation, tear or break	May need to interrupt foreplay, may dislodge during sex, allergy to rubber, inability to insert/remove, requires fitting by health care professional
Contraindications	None	None	None	None	Cervical dysplasia
Use effectiveness:	85%-95%, up to 98% is used with spermicide	80%-90%, up to 98% with spermicide	75%-90%	85%-90%	80%-90%; up to 98% with spermicide
Cost	$.25 - $2.00	$10-$25, additional spermicide and office visit	$1.00-2.50 each	$1.00-$2.50 each	$20-$25, additional spermicide and office visit

B.   Spermicides

Type:	Suppositories	Foam	Jelly, Cream	Film
Description/Name	Spermicide	Spermicide	Spermicide	Vaginal contraceptive film containing spermicide
Mechanism of Action	Chemical (nonoxynol-9 or octoxynol) to destroy the sperm; cell membrane so no viable sperm reach ovum	Chemical (nonoxynol-9 or octoxynol) to destroy the sperm, cell membrane so no viable sperm reach ovum	Chemical (nonoxynol-9 or octoxynol) to destroy the sperm, cell membrane so no viable sperm reach ovum	Chemical (nonoxynol-9) to destroy the sperm; cell membrane so no viable sperm reach ovum, place over cervix and wait to melt
Advantage	Over-the counter, some STD protection, easy to insert, adds lubrication, use along or with condom, good for a backup method if other method in question	Over-the counter, some STD protection, easy to insert, adds lubrication, use along or with condom, good for a backup method if other method in question	Over-the counter, some STD protection, easy to insert, adds lubrication, usually used with a diaphragm, good for a backup method if other method in question	Over-the counter, some STD protection, easy to insert, adds lubrication, use along or with condom, good for a backup method if other method in question

B. Spermicides (cont.)

Type:	Suppositories	Foam	Jelly, Cream	Film
Disadvantage (side effects)	Sensitivity to chemical, messy, short time of effectiveness so replace with each act of intercourse, short time to wait for dispersion	Sensitivity to chemical, messy, short time of effectiveness so replace with each act of intercourse, short time to wait for dispersion	Sensitivity to chemical, messy, short time of effectiveness so replace with each act of intercourse, short time to wait for dispersion	Sensitivity to chemical, messy, short time of effectiveness so replace with each act of intercourse, short time to wait for dispersion
Contraindication	Allergy, inability to correctly place	Allergy, inability to correctly place	Allergy, inability to correctly place	Allergy, inability to correctly place
Use effectiveness	80%-97%, increased with condom use	75%-97%, increased with condom use	75%-97%, increased with condom use	75%-97%, increased with condom use
Cost	$4-$10/package	$4-$10/package	$4-$10/package	$4-$10/package

C. Hormonal

Types:	Oral Contraceptive	Depomedroxyprogesterone Acetate	Norplant
Description	Combinations of estrogen (usually ethinyl estradiol) and progestins, dosages vary, progestin only pills available also	Depo-Provera, intramuscular progesterone injection	Levonorgestrel sub-epidermal implants in silicone capsules
Mechanism of Action	Prevent ovulation by suppression of gonadotropins, thicken cervical mucus, alter endometrium to prevent implantation, taken daily by mouth	Slow release to prevent ovulation, thicken cervical mucus, create thin, atrophic endometrium	Slow release of progestin to suppress ovulation and thicken cervical mucus, keeps endometrium thin and atrophic
Advantages	Doesn't interrupt sex, highly effective, decrease flow and cramps, regulates menses, protective against ovarian and endometrial cancer, may improve PMS, decreased PID, may suppress ovarian cyst formation, decrease benign breast tumors, premenopausal hormone replacement, easily reversible, may improve cholesterol profile	Injection of 150mg good for 3 months, already in place for sexual activity, decreased menses and cramps	Always in place for sexual activity, long-lasting - up to 5 years, rapid return to fertility after removal, no estrogen side effects, may have decreased cramps and menses

C.   Hormonal (cont.)

Types:	Oral Contraceptive	Depomedroxyprogesterone Acetate	Norplant
Disadvantages (side effects)	Must be remembered daily, no HIV protection, minor side effects (nausea, weight gain, breast tenderness, break through bleeding, etc.), circulatory complications/increased blood clots, benign liver tumors	Repeated injections, irregular bleeding, headaches, depression, nausea, breast tenderness, delayed return to fertility	Irregular menses, weight gain, no STD protection, trained professional for insertion and removal
Contraindications	Over 35 and a smoker, known clotting disorder/CVA/CAD, known estrogen dependent tumor, liver disease, pregnancy, unexplained vaginal bleeding, hypertension	Sensitivity to medication, unexplained vaginal bleeding	Sensitivity to levonorgestrel, liver disease, unexplained vaginal bleeding, thrombotic or CAD disease, pregnancy
Use effectiveness	99%	99%	99%
Cost	$20-$30/month, plus annual exam fee	$50-$100/shot, plus office visit	$350 for device plus office visit with insertion fee

D.   Intrauterine Device

Types:	Intrauterine Device
Description/Name	Plastic device placed in the uterine cavity, Paraguard and Progestasert only ones available in the United States
Mechanism of Action	To interfere with ova and sperm activity, fertilization and implantation, create local sterile inflammatory reaction. Exact mechanisms poorly understood, hormonal effects of progesterone in Progestasert
Advantages	Already in place without interrupting sexual activity, may decrease menses if contains progesterone
Disadvantages (side effects)	Possible increased menstrual flow and cramps, risk of pelvic infections, increase of ectopic pregnancy if pregnancy occurs, risk of displacement/spontaneous expulsion, uterine perforation, no STD protection
Contraindication	High risk factors for PID, desired fertility, anomalous uterine cavity, pregnancy, unexplained vaginal bleeding
Use effectiveness	94%-99%
Cost	$150-$400 including examination with insertion

E.   Sterilization

Types:	Female	Male
Description/Name	Tubal ligation, most common contraceptive method	Vasectomy
Mechanism of action	Blocking of fallopian tube by segment removal, cautery, clips, or Fallope rings to prevent sperm transport to meet ovum	Ligation of vas deferens to prevent sperm from leaving the testicle
Advantages	Permanent, highly effective, non-hormonal, no interruption of sexual activity	Permanent, highly effective, no interruption of sexual activity, office surgery with local anesthesia
Disadvantages (side effects)	Poorly reversible, requires anesthesia (all types), surgical risks of bleeding/infection/injury/anesthesia, no STD protection	Poorly reversible, surgical risks of bleeding/infection, no STD protection, majority develop sperm antibodies, recent concern of effect on prostate
Contraindication	Future fertility desired, not surgical candidate due to health risk	None
Types:	Female	Male
Use effectiveness	>99%	99%
Cost	$700-$1600	$125-$900

F.   Rhythm

Types:	Rhythm
Description/Name	Natural family planning, fertility awareness, periodic abstinence
Mechanism of Action	Avoid sex during fertile time in natural cycle. Identified by basal body temperature elevation, cervical mucus thinning, and calendar identification individual's ovulatory time
Advantages	No medications or devices involved, agrees with some religious beliefs
Disadvantages (side effects)	Requires dedication of patient to accurate record keeping, not good if natural cycles aren't regular especially early and late in reproductive years, no STD protection
Contraindications	None
Use effectiveness	80%-90% with practice and dedication
Cost	Nothing unless BBT thermometer bought

G.   Abortion

Types:	Abortion
Description/Name	Removal of the products of conception
Mechanism of Action	Surgically performed as a dilation and suction curettage, dilation and evacuation, hysterotomy or hysterectomy. Medically performed with prostaglandin E2, hypertonic saline or urea
Types	Abortion
Advantages	useful for implanted pregnancy up to 24 weeks
Disadvantages (side effects)	Surgical risks of infection, injury, bleeding, complications for future fertility, requires trained personnel
Contraindications	Pregnancy 24 weeks or greater
Cost effectiveness	99%
Cost	Varies - $250 and up

H.   Abstinence

Type:	Abstinence
Description/Name	None
Mechanism of Action	No sperm and egg contact
Advantages	No chance for STD's or pregnancy
Disadvantages (side effects)	Lack of intimacy
Contraindication	None
Use effectiveness	100%
Cost	Free

I.   Post-coital

Types:	Hormonal	Mechanical
Description/Name	"Morning After Pill", high dose combination oral contraceptive or ethinyl estradiol	IUD placement
Mechanism of Action	Luteolytic effect, out-of-phase endometrium, disordered tubal transport	Prevent implantation
Advantages	Useful if other method fails, after rape	Have 5-7 days to place, non-hormonal, can remain for continued contraception
Disadvantages (side effects)	Nausea, must be taken within 72 hours	All IUD complications, requires health care professional, not good method for anyone with infection risk
Contraindication	Similar to oral contraceptive	Desired pregnancy, abnormal uterine cavity
Use effectiveness	98%	>99%
Cost	$20-$30	$150-$400 for IUD and insertion

J.   Ineffective methods
      1.   Postcoital douching
      2.   Postcoital urination
      3.   Altered sexual positions
      4.   Coitus interruptus/withdrawal
      5.   Lactation

VAGINITIS AND VULVITIS

I.   Introduction

   A.   Vaginitis is a common complaint
      1.   Approximately 5 million office visits per year
      2.   Vaginitis is one of the top 25 reasons for physician visits

   B.   Vaginal itching and burning may be from a variety of causes
      1.   May be infectious, or non-infectious
      2.   May be confused with urinary complaints or GI complaints

   C.   "Vaginitis" or "yeast infection" may be the only term a patient knows for genital symptoms.

   D.   Complaints require a careful evaluation.

II.   Vaginitis

   A.   Normal Flora
      1.   Normally there are $10^5 - 10^7$ organisms per square centimeter of vaginal wall.

      2.   Predominate flora are usually Lactobacilli.

      3.   3-8 other species can usually be isolated by careful microbiology.
         a.   Group B streptococci 10-20%
         b.   *Mycoplasma hominis* 20-35%
         c.   *Ureaplasma urealyticum* 35-85%
         d.   *Gardnerella vaginalis* 40-60%
         e.   Bacteroides species 10-20%
         f.   *Peptococcus/peptostreptococcus* 6-10%
         g.   Anaerobic gram-positive rods 4-10%
         h.   Gram - negative aerobes 1- 2%

   B.   Normal vaginal secretions
      1.   Composed primarily of desquamated epithelial cells
      2.   Not visible at the introitus
      3.   Flocculent
      4.   White
      5.   Non-malodorous
      6.   pH 4.0 - 4.4

   C.   Evaluation of a patient with vaginitis
      1.   History
         a.   Itching
         b.   Burning, pain
         c.   Discharge - amount, color, odor
         d.   Dyspareunia - location (introital, vaginal, pelvic/lower abdomen), severity

e. Duration of symptoms
f. Previous episodes
g. Previous therapies
h. Underlying medical conditions - diabetes, pregnancy, immune suppression antibiotic used.
i. Sexual history
j. Self - therapy

2. Physical examination
a. Vulvar lesions or inflammation
b. Presence of discharge at introitus
c. Character of vaginal discharge

3. Laboratory evaluation
a. Saline mount - evaluate for Trichomonads, "clue" cells, evaluate for white Blood cells, squamous cells.
b. KOH preparation - use 10% KOH, evaluate for fungal forms
c. Vaginal pH - Normal < 4.5, pH > 4.5 indicates bacterial vaginosis or *Trichomonas*.
d. Whiff test - odor is released on addition of 10% KOH, foul or fishy odor indicates bacterial vaginosis; "Yeasty" odor indicates fungal infection
e. Gram stain - direct smear from vagina
f. Cultures - rarely indicated except in difficult or recurrent cases. If done, MUST be done in a quantitative manner. If done, MUST be done separately for anaerobes, aerobes fungi and trichomonads with appropriate transfer media. If done, MUST have a microbiology lab capable of isolating and identifying aerobes, anaerobes, trichomonads and fungi.

D. Common types of vaginitis
1. Bacterial vaginosis
a. Alteration in the normal flora; decline in numbers of lactobacilli; overgrowth of gardnerella and anaerobes
b. Diagnosis - by wet mount with "Clue" cells and minimal WBC's; cultures; Whiff test.
c. Therapy - metronidazole, clindamycin vaginal gel

2. Description of fungal vaginitis -
a. Usually *Candida* species
b. Diagnosis - KOH prep; special cultures
c. Therapy - over the counter anti fungals, boric acid vaginal tablets

3. Description of trichomonas -
a. Flagellated protozoan producing yellow green discharge, some itching and odor may be present.
b. Diagnosis - wet mount, gram stain
c. Therapy - metronidazole

III. **Vulvitis**

    A.   Evaluation of a patient with vulvitis

        1.   History

            a.   Nature, duration, location of symptoms

            b.   Previous diagnosis and therapy

        2.   Physical examination

            a.   Gross examination

            b.   Colposcopy may be helpful

            c.   Wash with dilute acetic acid to find hyperkeratotic lesions

            d.   Stain with toluidine blue to find hyperplasia

        3.   Laboratory evaluation

            a.   Cultures of ulcers for herpes virus

            b.   Biopsy of suspected lesions

    B.   Common types of vulvitis

        1.   Fungal

        2.   Vulvar dystropies

            a.   Lichen sclerosis

            b.   Hyperplastic dystrophy

            c.   Vulvar intraepithelial neoplasia

        3.   Atrophic

            a.   Due to lack of estrogen

            b.   Thin, atrophic skin

            c.   Symptoms - itching, burning

        4.   Allergic/irritant

        5.   Vestibular adenitis/vulvar vestibulitis

            a.   Rare syndrome characterized by intense tenderness and burning of the vulvar vestibule.

            b.   Physical findings limited to vestibular erythema of varying degree.

            c.   Biopsy shows non-specific chronic inflammation.

        6.   Human papilloma virus - condyloma acuminata

        7.   Paget's disease

        8.   Pudendal neuralgia

IV.   Sequelae of Vaginitis/Vulvitis

A.   Most episodes respond to therapy with no sequelae

B.   Sexual dysfunction
1.   Inhibited sexual desire
2.   Vaginismus

C.   Other infectious sequelae
1.   Pelvic inflammatory disease
2.   Intra-amniotic infection
3.   Post partum endometritis
4.   Premature delivery

PAP SMEARS AND BENIGN CERVICAL DISEASE

I. **Pap Smears**

    A.   Screening test for cervical cel abnormalities

    B.   Recommended by age 18 or onset of sexual activity

    C.   Has reduced incidence of cervical cancer by detecting precancerous lesions

II. **Technique**

    A.   Ectocervical scraping with a spatula first

    B.   Endocervical sampling with an endocervical brush
        1.   In pregnancy, this is replaced with a moistened cotton-tipped swab

    C.   Both samples are placed on a glass slide and fixed with formalin or alcohol within 15 seconds to prevent air-drying artifact

    D.   Best performed when there is no infection, menses, medications or lubricants present

III. **Accuracy**

    A.   False negative range 15-40%

    B.   Usually due to sampling errors

    C.   May be affected by age, contraceptive method, pregnancy, or prior cervical surgery

IV. **Risk Factors for Cervical Dysplasia**

    A.   Multiple sex partners

    B.   Early age of first intercourse (< 18)

    C.   History of STD's - especially HPV

    D.   DES exposure

    E.   Uncircumcised partner

    F.   Smoking

V. Reporting Results

A. Old systems include
   1. Class system
   2. Dysplasia degree system
   3. CIN (cervical intraepithelial neoplasia) system

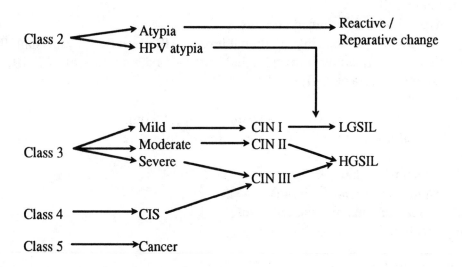

B. Currently accepted is the Bethesda System

BETHESDA SYSTEM FOR CERVICAL/VAGINAL CYTOLOGY

<u>Adequacy of Specimen</u>
- satisfactory for evaluation
- satisfactory for evaluation but limited by.............
- unsatisfactory for evaluation................(give reason)

<u>General Category</u> (optional)
- within normal limits
- benign cellular changes
- epithelial cell abnormality

<u>Descriptive Diagnosis</u>
- Benign cellular changes
  - Infection
    - Trichomonas vaginalis
    - Fungal organisms
    - Coccobacilli predominance
    - Actinomyces

- Herpes simplex virus
- Other
  - Reactive changes
    - inflammatory
    - atrophy
    - radiation
    - IUD
    - other

<u>Epithelial cell abnormalities</u>
- Squamous cell
  - atypical of undetermined etiology
  - low-grade squamous intraepithelial lesion - HPV and mild dysplasia/CINI
  - high-grade squamous intraepithelial lesion - moderate dysplasia/CINII, severedysplasia and CIS/CINIII
- Glandular cell
  - normal endometrial cells in a postmenopausal women
  - atypical glandular cells of undetermined significance
  - endocervical adenocarcinoma
  - endometrial adenocarcinoma
  - extrauterine adenocarcinoma
  - adenocarcinoma not otherwise specified
- Other malignant neoplasm's - specify

Hormonal evaluation

VI.   Methods to Evaluate Dysplasia

A.   Colposcopy with directed biopsies - standard Tx

B.   Random biopsies

C.   Schiller's test - iodine staining (Lugol's)

D.   Cervicography - 35mm photo through colposcope

E.   Indications for colposcopy
1.   Pap with any degree of dysplasia
2.   Grossly abnormal cervix
3.   Persistent squamous atypia

Abnormal Cytology

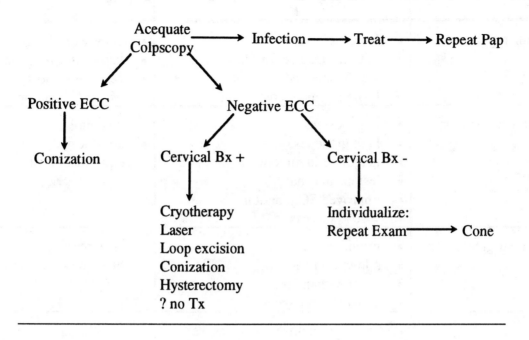

VII. Technique of Colposcopy

A. Speculum placed with the Pap, repeated as needed. Acetic Acid 3-5% is applied to the cervix. Abnormalities of color, surface contour, and vascular pattern are evaluated. Biopsies are taken of abnormal areas. The endocervical canal is sampled with an endocervical curette. Hemostatic solutions are applied as needed. All of the transformation zone must be seen.

B. Treatment options
1. Based on the examination and the biopsy results

CERVICAL DYSPLASIA
TREATMENT OPTIONS

	PRO	CON
Cryotherapy	<ul><li>No anesthesia</li><li>minimal chance for bleeding</li><li>> 90% success</li><li>low equipment cost</li></ul>	<ul><li>watery discharge</li><li>vasomotor reaction</li><li>cervical stenosis</li><li>poor SC junction</li></ul>
Laser Vaporization	<ul><li>large lesions</li><li>high grade lesions</li><li>glandular involvement</li><li>lesions in canal</li><li>improved SC junction</li><li>> 90% success</li></ul>	<ul><li>bleeding</li><li>anesthesia?</li><li>equipment cost</li></ul>
Electrosurgical Loop	<ul><li>provides specimen</li><li>allows conization</li><li>cheaper than laser</li><li>won't ablate cancer</li></ul>	<ul><li>anesthesia?</li><li>bleeding</li></ul>
Conization	<ul><li>evaluates endocervical disease</li><li>cure rate > 98% with negative margins</li><li>avoids hysterectomy</li><li>evaluates invasion</li><li>knife or laser</li></ul>	<ul><li>anesthesia needed</li><li>bleeding in 5-10%</li><li>infertility</li><li>incompetent cervix</li></ul>
Hysterectomy	<ul><li>definite therapy</li></ul>	<ul><li>increased morbidity and mortality</li></ul>

PELVIC RELAXATION

I. Definition:

A. Disorders of pelvic support structures.
1. Includes cystocele, rectocele, enterocele, urethrocele and uterine prolapse.
2. Involves levator ani muscles and endopelvic fascia.

II. Predisposing Factors

A. Obesity

B. Childbirth

C. Smoking/chronic cough

D. Age, estrogen deficiency

E. Repeated/long term lifting

F. Trauma

II. Symptoms

A. Pelvic/vaginal pressure or fullness

B. Stress urinary incontinence

C. Straining or digitalization with bowel movement

D. Backache

E. Dysparunia

F. Occasional urinary urgency, feeling of incomplete voiding

III. Examination

A. Urethrocele
1. Bulge in lower third of the anterior vaginal wall underlying the urethra.
2. Pressure applied may cause a small amount of urine to be expelled

B. Cystocele
1. Bulge in anterior vaginal wall of varying degrees.
2. Usually described by extent of prolapse in relation to introitus

C. Rectocele
1. Bulge of posterior vaginal wall into vagina.
2. Most evident with valsalva. Rectovaginal exam can help confirm its extent

D. Enterocele
1. Hernia of vaginal apex through pouch of Douglas.
2. Includes peritoneum and small bowel.
3. Most common after hysterectomy

E. Procidentia
1. Prolapse of the uterus. Described by degrees
   a. First degree: into upper vagina
   b. Second degree: lower vagina to introitus
   c. Third degree: through introitus

IV. Nonsurgical Treatments

A. Pessary
1. Usually a Smith Hodge.
2. Can be used for all types of relaxation

B. Kegel
1. Exercises levator ani muscles.
2. May be performed with vaginal cones but are usually done without

C. Estrogen
1. Will help improve integrity of vaginal tissues

V. Surgical Therapies

A. Urethrocele
1. Anterior colporrhaphy performed which will include repair of the usually accompanying cystocele.
2. Sutures are placed in the pubocervical fascia at the level of the urethrovesical junction (bladder neck) and continued along the urethra where the urethrocele is present

B. Cystocele
1. Anterior colporrhaphy is performed to imbricate the pubocervical fascia over the bladder

C. Rectocele
1. A posterior colporrhaphy is performed to approximate the perirectal fascia, which includes portions of the levator ani muscles, over the rectum.
2. Often a perineorrhaphy is also performed to correct vaginal outlet relaxation.

D.   Enterocele
   1.   May be performed abdominally or vaginally, sometimes in conjunction with other reparative procedures.
   2.   The peritoneal sac is separated from other tissue and ligated at its neck.
   3.   Obliteration of the cul-de-sac may be accomplished by plicating the uterosacral ligaments or pursestring sutures of the endopelvic fascia. This will help prevent recurrence.

E.   Uterine Prolapse
   1.   A vaginal or abdominal hysterectomy should be performed.
   2.   Almost always an anterior and posterior colporrhaphy will also be needed.
   3.   A colpocleisis may be done which adheres the anterior and posterior vaginal walls with or without a uterus present above the closure.

URINARY INCONTINENCE

I.   Definition:

    A.   When involuntary loss of urine is a social or hygienic problem and one that can be objectively demonstrated.

    B.   Involves approximately 10% of women.

II. **Types**

    A.   Stress
        1.   Definition
            a.   An involuntary and immediate loss of urine when intravesical pressure exceeds urethral pressure. Occurs with increased intra-abdominal pressure and in the absence of detrusor activity.
            b.   May include 75%-80% of incontinence problems

        2.   Predisposing factors
            a.   Pregnancy and delivery
            b.   Obesity
            c.   Chronic cough
            d.   Heavy lifting and frequent straining (similar to pelvic relaxation causes)

        3.   Symptoms
            a.   Urine leakage with cough, sneeze, laugh, lifting, and often certain exercise activities

        4.   Anatomic defect - lowered urethral resistance due to displacement of the urethra and urethrovesical junction away from the pubic bone and out of the abdominal cavity

        5.   Diagnosis - demonstration of urine with valsalva and in the absence of detrusor activity

        6.   Treatment - ideally surgical with the goal of returning the proximal urethra to an intra-abdominal position and supporting the bladder base. Possible post-operative complications include the temporary inability to void spontaneously and osteitis pubis (1%) following retropubic urethropexies
            a.   Non-surgical
                1)   Kegel exercises (pubococcygeal)
                2)   Estrogen therapy
                3)   Bladder training (voiding schedule)
                4)   Biofeedback
                5)   Medications

        b.   Surgical
             1)   Anterior colporrhaphy/Kelly
             2)   Plication
             3)   Burch
             4)   Pereyra
             5)   Sling
             6)   Other variations

B.   Urge

1.   Definition - also called bladder instability. Includes from 10-30% of incontinence problems, but percentage increases with age. Majority of patients (90%) are neurologically normal

    a.   Types
        1)   Motor - uninhibited detrusor contractions
        2)   Sensory - due to strong sensory input from bladder. No uninhibited detrusor activity

2.   Predisposing factors - motor type is usually of unknown etiology, but may be upper motor neuron lesion. Sensory often due to inflammation, mechanical irritation, neoplastic or hormonal epithelial changes, and radiation

3.   Symptoms
    a.   Motor has uninhibited loss of small mounts of urine, nocturia, frequency
    b.   Sensory can inhibit contractions and may have discomfort with bladder filling

4.   Anatomic defect - none except bladder mucosal changes with some causes of sensory urge incontinence

5.   Diagnosis - cystometry reveals uninhibited bladder contraction > 15 cm of water, opening of vesical neck with a detrusor contraction

6.   Treatment - treat identifiable cause, i.e., bladder infection, removal of stone, add estrogen; otherwise, use pharmacological therapy to include anticholinergics, alpha-adrenergics, imipramine Hcl, and others. Also voiding schedules, biofeedback and surgical means

C.   Overflow

1.   Definition - a problem of urinary retention (overdistension) with intravesical pressure exceeding maximum urethral pressure.
    a.   Not associated with detrusor activity.
    b.   Usually associated with residuals > 150 cc.
    c.   Sometimes called neurogenic bladder

2.   Predisposing factors
    a.   Neurologic disease
    b.   CNS trauma or tumors
    c.   Medications
    d.   Peripheral neuropathies
    e.   Obstruction

3. Symptoms
    a. Voiding small amounts
    b. Feeling of incomplete emptying
    c. Leaking small amounts

4. Anatomic defect
    a. May be none
    b. Possible obstruction of urethra

5. Diagnosis
    a. High residual urine volume
    b. Cystoscopy revealing obstruction

6. Treatment - treat any medical illnesses as much as possible, relieve obstruction. May learn self-catheterization

D. Extraurethral
1. Definition - loss of urine other than through the urethra

2. Predisposing factors
    a. Surgery
    b. Congenital anomalies
    c. Radiation therapy

3. Symptoms - constant small amounts of urine loss sometimes confused with vaginal discharge

4. Anatomic defect
    a. Fistula
    b. Ectopic ureter
    c. Urethral diverticula

5. Diagnosis
    a. Dye studies for leakage site
    b. Cystoscopy
    c. IVP
    d. Urethroscopy

6. Treatment - repair of anatomical defect

III. Initial Evaluation

A. Genito-urinary history
1. Specifics of incontinence
    a. Duration
    b. Frequency
    c. Dysuria
    d. Precipitating factors
    e. Hematuria
    f. Enuresis
    g. Urgency

2.   Medical diseases
3.   Medications
4.   Surgeries
5.   Social/occupational

B.   Initial examination
    1.   Evaluate
        a.   Pelvic support loss
        b.   Estrogen status
        c.   Bimanual examination
        d.   Neurologic deficits (S2-S4)
        e.   Urine culture
    2.   Test
        a.   Supine or upright urine leakage with valsalva and full bladder
        b.   Q-tip test - document urethrovesical junction mobility - hypermobility if change > 35
        c.   Bonney test - elevates urethrovesical junction with fingers
        d.   Pessary test - elevates urethrovesical junction without occlusion of the urethra. Use Smith-Hodge pessary

C.   Additional testing
    1.   Cystoscopy - visualized bladder mucosa, urethra and sphincter for abnormalities such as inflammation, fistula, diverticula, foreign body, urethrovesical junction function and mobility

    2.   Urodynamics - measures relationship between bladder pressure and volume. a.Especially useful for demonstration of uninhibited detrusor contractions
        b.   May use single or multichannel system
        c.   Fill bladder with sterile water, saline, CO_2, urine or dye
        d.   Fill at rates between 10-100 ml/min, often in 50 ml increments
        e.   Record pressures at rest, first desure (150cc), urgent need, maximum pressure (500 cc) and bladder capacity (300-500 cc) of water
        f.   Normal rise in pressure, 10-15 cm water
        g.   Note presence and frequency of detrusor contractions
        h.   Use provocative measures to make test highly predictive
        i.   Check residual after patient empties bladder

    3.   Uroflowometry - obtains average urine flow rate.
        a.   Normal >20 ml/sec.
        b   Normal voiding is complete in 20 seconds

$$\frac{\text{volume of urine}}{\text{length of time voiding}} = \text{average flow rate}$$

    4.   Video cystourethrogram - uses fluoroscopy to view bladder function in comparison with pressures

SEXUALLY TRANSMITTED DISEASES

I. Gonorrhea

Organism	*Neisseria gonorrhea*, gram negative diplococcal bacteria
Transmission	Direct contact with infected mucus membranes (urethra, cervix, anus, throat or eyes); prefers endocervix
Incubation	2-10 days
Signs/symptoms	Mucopurulent discharge form vagina, urethra, or anus; dysuria; may be exacerbated after menses; pharyngitis, abnormal uterine bleeding
Duration	Until treated
Diagnosis	Culture on Thayer-martin agar, gram stain with gram negative intracellular diplococci
Treatment	Ceftriaxone 250 mg IM, Cefixime 400 mg po, Ciprofloxin 500 mg po, or Ofloxacin 400 mg po for one dose. Should always treat for chlamydia
Complications	Upper genital tract infections (PID), sterility, disseminated infection to include arthritis, endocarditis; perihepatitis (Fitz-Hugh-Curtis syndrome), transmission to newborn

II. Chlamydia

Organism	*Chlamydia trachomatis*, obligate intracellular parasite
Transmission	Direct contact with infected mucus membranes
Incubation	7 - 14 days
Signs/symptoms	Vaginal discharge from mucopurulent cervicitis, dysuria, most common bacterial STD, often asymptomatic
Duration	Until treated
Diagnosis	Tissue culture PCR immuno assays
Treatment	Doxycycline 100 mg po bid x 7-10 days, Azithromycin 2 mg po Erythromycin base 500 mg qid x 7 days, EES 800 mg po quid x 7 days, Ofloxacin 300 po bid x 7 days, Sulfisoxazole 500 mg po quid x 10 days
Complications	Upper genital tract infection (PID), sterility, infections to newborn, non-gonococcal urethritis, epididymitis

III. Herpes

Organism	Herpes simplex virus, DNA virus types 1 and 2
Transmission	Direct contact with blister or open sore
Incubation	3-7 days, but variable

Signs/symptoms	Vesicles, usually multiple, that rupture to form painful, open ulcers. Primary infection involves flu-like symptoms. Virus remains dormant in nerve root. May have prodrome of burning, pain or tingling
Duration	12 days primary, 4.5 days recurrent; recurrent outbreaks at varying intervals
Diagnosis	Tissue culture of serous secretions in blisters or ulcers, cytologic stain showing multinucleated giant cells with intranuclear inclusions. Fluorescent antibody can detect type
Treatment	No cure; treatment with Acyclovir may decrease outbreaks
Complications	Neuralgia, urethral strictures, increased risk of cervical cancer, neonatal infection during delivery, fetal wastage

IV.   Condyloma Acuminata (Genital warts)

Organism	Human papilloma virus, DNA virus causing epithelial infections
Transmission	Direct sexual contact with warts, vertical transmission from mother to neonate
Incubation	one to many months
Signs/symptoms	Painless warty growths on genitals, perineum, vagina, cervix; may have local irritation or itching, most common symptomatic viral STD
Duration	Remain unless treated, HPV never completely eradicated with 80% recurrence rate
Diagnosis	Visually, can be biopsied or varityped for DNA, suggested by Pap
Treatment	Cryotherapy, podophyllin, Trichloracetic acid, laser, electrosurgical excision, surgical removal, 5-fluorouracil, interferon
Complications	Increase risk of cervical and vulvar cancer; growths may become large enough to obstruct vagina, rectum, throat; neonatal laryngeal papillomas

V.   Syphilis

Organism	*Treponema pallidum*, an anaerobic spirochete
Transmission	Direct contact with rash or sore
Incubation	Average 3 weeks (10-90 days)
Signs/symptoms	*Primary:* single, painless, indurated chancre sore (ulcer) at the site of entry *Secondary:* skin rash or mucus patches, lymphadenopathy, condyloma lata *Tertiary:* asymptomatic but includes involvement of other organ systems *Latent:* patients are without signs of symptoms
Duration	Chancre present 3-6 weeks without treatment, secondary 2-6 weeks

Diagnosis		*Primary:* clinical presentation with typical lesions, examination of organisms from lesion by darkfield exam, newly positive serology or 4-fold increase in titer, or known exposure within 90 days of lesion
		Secondary: clinical presentation, demonstration of organism from lesion, positive serology - fluorescent antibody techniques (FTA)
		Tertiary: clinical presentation with CNS, cardiovascular, etc. involvement
		Latent: no clinical signs but positive serology causes suspicion

Diagnosis — *Primary:* clinical presentation with typical lesions, examination of organisms from lesion by darkfield exam, newly positive serology or 4-fold increase in titer, or known exposure within 90 days of lesion
Secondary: clinical presentation, demonstration of organism from lesion, positive serology - fluorescent antibody techniques (FTA)
Tertiary: clinical presentation with CNS, cardiovascular, etc. involvement
Latent: no clinical signs but positive serology causes suspicion

Treatment — Primary, secondary or <1 year duration - Benzathine Penicillin 2.4 million units. More than 1 year duration   2.4 million units IM q week for 3 weeks
Penicillin allergic: Doxycycline 100 mg bid for 15-30 days depending on duration
Erythromycin 500 mg qid for 2 weeks if unable to take other medications

Complications — Brain damage, heart disease, congenital defects to fetus, gumma formation

VI. Human Immunodeficiency Virus

Organism — Human Immunodeficiency Virus, RNA virus

Transmission — Contact with infected body fluids, sharing needles, blood transfusion

Incubation — Months to years

Signs/symptoms — Fatigue, lymphadenopathy, weight loss, cough, diarrhea, night sweats

Duration — No cure, treat symptomes

Diagnosis — HIV antibodies in blood; ELISA test, Western blot; presence of pathognomonic infections such as Kaposi's sarcoma, pneumocystis pneumonia

Treatment — Treat symptoms and infections as needed. Zidovudine (AZT)

Complications — Opportunistic infections, death

VII. Chancroid

Organism — *Haemophilus ducreyi*, gram negative bacillus

Transmission — Sexual; especially labia, clitoris, and posterior fourchette, often at sites traumatized during sex

Incubation — 3-5 days

Signs/symptoms — One to few painful pustules becoming ulcers surrounded by erythema, may be necrotic and purulent; often has painful unilateral inguinal adenopathy and may develop inguinal bubo

Duration — Weeks

Diagnosis — Cultures difficult; clinical; gram stain with rods in chain

Treatment	Ceftriaxone 250 mg IM, Erythromycin 500 mg po qid x 10 days, Azithromycin 1 gm po, Ampicillin-Cavulanate 500/125 mg po tid x 7 days, Ciprofloxacin 500 mg po bid x 7 days
Complications	Fistula, secondary infection of lesions

VIII. Lymphogranuloma Venereum

Organism	*Chlamydia trachomatis*, serotypes L1, L2, L3
Transmission	Sexual
Incubation	4-21 days
Signs/symptoms	Inguinal lymphadenopathy which may progress to abscess; single non-painful vesicle or ulcer followed in 1-4 weeks by inguinal lymphadenopathy which may progress to abscess. Groove sign of inguinal ligament; systemic symptoms, proctitis
Duration	Days
Diagnosis	Clinical; LGV compliment fixation test for antibody titers; tissue culture; monoclonal antibodies; especially in tropical areas; Frei intradermal test for previous infections
Treatment	Doxycycline 100 mg po bid x 21 days, also can use 500 mg Erythromycin 500 mg po qid x 21 days. Aspirate abscesses
Complications	Dissemination with nephropathy, hepatomegaly, or phlebitis; perianal abscess, fistula, local edema

IX. Trichomonas Vaginalis

Organism	Protozoan
Transmission	Sexually transmitted vaginal infection
Incubation	None
Signs/symptoms	Yellow-green vaginal discharge, possible pruritus; "strawberry" cervix
Duration	Until treated
Diagnosis	Wet mount with motile flagellated protozoans, may be picked up on pap smear
Treatment	Metronidazole given either 2 gm po/500 mg po bid x 7 days, 250 mg po tid x 7 days
Complications	Continued vaginal discharge

X. Granuloma Inguinale

Organism	*Calymmato-bacterium granulomatis* (Donovanosis), gram negative
Transmission	Sexual, can spread by autoinoculation

Incubation	8-12 weeks
Signs/symptoms	Single or multiple subcutaneous nodules which become eroded, painless, granulomatous ulcers
Diagnosis	Donovan bodies in microscopic specimens from lesions, clinical presentation
Treatment	Tetracycline 500 mg po qid for 21 days or until resolution
Complications	Secondary infections of lesions, scarring of lesion sites

DYSMENORRHEA

I. **Definition: painful menstruation**

II. **Incidence: approximately 60-70%**

III. **Types**

    A.   Primary

        1.   Etiology - thought due to excess prostaglandin F2alpha from the secretory endometrium causing smooth muscle stimulation, not due to organic causes

        2.   Symptoms

            a.   Lower abdominal cramps especially during first 2 days of menses which may radiate to back

            b.   Nausea

            c.   Vomiting

            d.   Diarrhea

            e.   Fatigue

            f.   Headache

            g.   Usually begins once cycles become ovulatory in early reproductive years and cycles are regular

        3.   Signs - increased intrauterine pressures

        4.   Examination

            a.   Normal

            b.   Performed to rule out secondary causes

        5.   Laboratory - None

        6.   Treatment

            a.   Non-steroidal anti-inflammatory medications

            b.   Oral contraceptives

    B.   Secondary (acquired)

        1.   Etiology - identifiable organic cause

            a.   Leiomyoma

            b.   Adenomyosis

            c.   Polyps

            d.   Endometriosis (#1)

            e.   IUD's

            f.   Infection

            g.   Ovarian cysts

            h.   Adhesions

            i.   Congenital anomalies

            j.   Cervical stenosis

            k.   Stress/psychogenic

2. Symptoms - depend on etiology. Usually begins in mid to later reproductive years (after 20)
   a. Dysparunia
   b. Menorrhagia
   c. Fever

3. Signs
   a. Pelvic mass
   b. Fixed uterus
   c. Uterosacral nodularity
   d. Purulent cervical discharge

4. Examination - exclude
   a. Uterine enlargement
   b. Adnexal masses
   c. Cervical anomalies

5. Laboratory
   a. Ultrasound
   b. CBC

6. Treatment - directed towards etiology; may be medical including:
   a. Non-steroidal anti-inflammatory medications
   b. Oral contraceptives
   c. Antibiotics
   d. GnRH agonists
   e. May be surgical via laparoscopy or laparotomy to remove:
      1. Adnexal cysts/masses
      2. Hysterectomy
      3. Oophorectomy
      4. Correction of anomaly such as imperforate hymen, hysteroscopy, hysterosalpingogram, D&C

PELVIC INFLAMMATORY DISEASE

I. **Definition:**

    A.   Infection and inflammation of the upper genital tract.

    B.   Includes endometritis, salpingitis, peritonitis and tubo-ovarian abscess.

II. **Incidence:**

    A.   1-2% of sexually active females per year.

    B.   85% spontaneous and 15% secondary to interruption of cervical mucus barrier (Endometrial biopsy, D&C, hysteroscopy, IUD insertion).

III. **Risk Factors:**

    A.   Teenagers

    B.   Multiple sexual partners

    C.   Frequent intercourse

    D.   Excessive douching

    E.   No contraception

    F.   Recent pelvic procedure

    G.   Prior pelvic infection

    H.   Poor socioeconomic status

IV. **Organisms:**

    A.   Majority are polymicrobial infections,

    B.   More than 99% are ascending infections from the vagina or cervix.

    C.   Remaining are from local spread of other intra-abdominal process (appendix, abscess) or possible hematogenous or lymphatic spread.

    D.   Sexually transmitted:
        1.   Neisseria gonorrhea
        2.   Chlamydia trachomatis
        3.   Mycoplasma hominis

E.   Endogenous Aerobic:
    1.   Nonhemolytic streptococcus
    2.   *Escherichia coli*
    3.   *B* hemolytic streptococci
    4.   Coagulase negative streptococci

F.   Endogenous anaerobes:
    1.   Bacteroides
    2.   Peptostreptococcus
    3.   Peptococcus

V.   **Signs and Symptoms: (Most common to less common)**

A.   Pelvic pain

B.   Adnexal tenderness or mass

C.   Purulent vaginal discharge

D.   Elevated erythrocyte sedimentation rate (ESR)

E.   Irregular vaginal bleeding

F.   Fever >38 C

G.   Urinary symptoms

H.   Nausea and vomiting

VI.   **Diagnostic Testing: History and Examination - Best Information**

A.   Human chorionic gonadotropin - rule out pregnancy

B.   ESR - nonspecific indicator of inflammation

C.   CBC - WBC elevated in about 10% cervical cultures

D.   Ultrasound - for masses/abscess

E.   Culdocentesis - for blood or pus

F.   Laparoscopy - gold standard for definitive diagnosis; finds about 25% normal pelvic structures

G.   Endometrial biopsy - for endometritis

VII. **Differential Diagnosis**

    A.   Appendicitis

    B.   Endometriosis

    C.   Hemorrhagic corpus luteum

    D.   Ectopic pregnancy

    E.   Benign ovarian tumor

    F.   Adhesions

    G.   Chronic salpingitis/hydrosalpinx

    H.   Ovarian torsion

    I.   Ruptured ovarian cyst

VIII. **Management**

    A.   Goals
        1.   Resolution of infection and its symptoms
        2.   Preservation of tubal function

    B.   Treat the male partner when possible.

    C.   Decide if inpatient vs. outpatient treatment is needed. Hospitalize if:
        1.   Nulliparous
        2.   Tubo-ovarian abscess/compile present
        3.   Failed outpatient therapy
        4.   Evidence of non-pelvic peritonitis
        5.   Uncertain diagnosis
        6.   GI symptoms - nausea/vomiting
        7   Recent operative or diagnostic procedure
        8.   IUD present
        9.   Pregnant
        10.   Adolescent/teenagers

    D.   Outpatient antibiotic regimens include one of the following and a return visit in 2-3 days:
        1.   Ceftriaxone 250 mg IM
        2.   Cefoxitin 2 gm IM plus 1gm probenecid po
        3.   Equivalent cephalosporin along with one of the following
            a.   Doxycycline 100 mg po bid for 10-14 days
            b.   Tetracycline hydrochloride 500 mg po 4x daily for 10-14 days

       c.   Erythromycin 500 mg po qid for 10-14 days (if unable to tolerate tetracyclines).

       d.   Azithromycin 2 gm po, Ofloxacin 300 mg bid x10 days

E.   Inpatient antibiotic regimens include one of the following:

     1.   Doxycycline 100 mg IV bid with cefoxitin 2 gm IV qid. Continue until clinically improved 48 hours. Complete 10-14 days total doxycycline with oral medication.

     2.   Clindamycin 900 mg IV tid with gentamicin 2 mg/kg loading dose IV then 1.5 mg/kg q8 hours. Continue until clinically improved 48 hours. Complete 10-14 days total with clindamycin 450 mg po qid or doxycycline 100 mg po bid.

     3.   Cefotetan 2 gm IV q 12 hours with doxycycline 100 mg IV bid until clinically improved 48 hours. Complete 10-14 days total with doxycycline po.

IX.   Complications: **25% experience sequelae to include:**

A.   Ectopic pregnancies - due to tubal damage

B.   Chronic pelvic pain - adhesions, hydrosalpinx, dysparunia

C.   Infertility - tubal damage, paraovarian adhesions. Increases with each episode of infection

D.   Increased chance for reinfection - may be due to mucosal damage vs. reinfection

E.   Perihepatitis - Fitz-Hugh-Curtis syndrome develops in 5-10%

F.   Pelvic abscess - about 10% of acute PID; bilateral more than half the time; require surgery 50% of the time due to lack of resolution 2-3 weeks after antibiotics

G.   Death - usually due to ruptured TOA's

UTERINE LEIOMYOMAS

I. **Definition** - A benign tumor originating from smooth muscle cells. Sometimes called fibroids or myomas. Contain varying amounts of fibrous tissue which is probably degenerated smooth muscle cells.

II. **Facts**
- A. Most during fifth decade
- B. Most frequent pelvic tumor
- C. Usually multiple
- D. Most common pelvic site is uterine corpus
- E. Found in 25% of white women and 50% of black women
- F. Growth probably stimulated by estrogen
- G. Grow by pushing borders with a pseudocapsule

III. **Locations**
- A. Subserosal - located under the outer serosal surface of the uterus
- B. Intramural - within the muscular wall of the uterus; also called interstitial
- C. Submucosal - under the endometrium. Symptoms especially bleeding and cramping
- D. Intraligamentary - within the broad ligament. Easy to confuse with adnexal masses
- E. Pedunculated - attached by a pedicle. May originate from serosal or mucosal locations
- F. Parasitic - usually pedunculated myoma that obtain an alternative blood supply other than the uterus
- G. Cervical - located in the cervix instead of uterine corpus

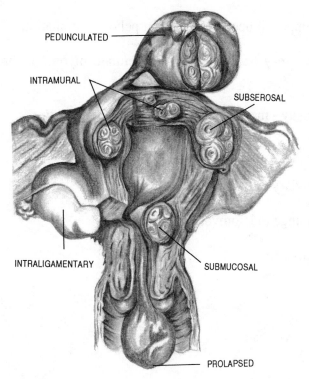

IV.   Appearance

    A.   Gross - uterus may appear smooth but enlarged or grossly nodular. Cut surface is pearl-white and glistening. Base of pedicel has major blood supply

    B.   Histologically - proliferation of smooth muscle cells in bundles. Fibrous connective tissue between bundles

V.   Symptoms

    A.   Pelvic pressure

    B.   Urinary frequency

    C.   Pain - dysmenorrhea, Dysparunia, abnormal uterine bleeding

    D.   Infertility

    E.   Pregnancy complications - preterm labor, abortion, dystocia

    F.   May be asymptomatic

VI.   Diagnosis

    A.   Suggested by history

    B.   Bimanual examination - often confirmatory

    C.   Pelvic ultrasound - if needed to support pelvic examination

    D.   Laparoscopy - may be needed to differentiate myoma in broad ligament from adnexal mass

    E.   Abdominal x-ray - may identify myoma with calcifications

VII.   Complications

    A.   Anemia secondary to menorrhagia

    B.   Neoplastic change to leiomyosarcoma (< 1%)

    C.   Polycythemia - rare

    D.   Hydroureter

VIII. **Degeneration - occurs when blood supply can no longer reach center of myoma**

    A.   Hyaline - 65% - most common. An acellular type of change that occurs slowly

    B.   Myxomatous - 15%

    C.   Calcific - 10% - common in larger myomas, older women

    D.   Cystic - liquefaction

    E.   Fatty

    F.   Red/necrotic/carneous - acute from of degeneration. Often occurs in pregnancy due to rapid growth beyond ability of blood supply. May become secondarily infected. Associated with acute pain

    G.   Sarcomatous - rare malignant degeneration, < 1%

IX. **Treatment**

    A.   Hormonal
        1.   Progesterone - given to reduce estrogen levels
        2.   GnRH agonist - creates menopausal situation by stopping gonadotropin stimulation of menstrual cycle. This decreases estrogen production and its stimulation to tumor growth. Used preoperatively to decrease myoma size

    B.   Surgical
        1.   Myomectomy - removal of individual fibroids - usually with plans with preserving fertility
        2.   Hysterectomy - removal of the uterus and involved fibroids when fertility no longer desired. Often performed when the uterus attains the size of a 14 week pregnancy due to difficulty in evaluation of the adnexa

    C.   Observation - If asymptomatic and less than 14 week size, may observe. Intervene if rapid growth occurs (concern for sarcomatous change) or symptoms begin

ENDOMETRIOSIS

I. **Definition:** presence of endometrial glands and stroma in locations outside of the uterine cavity.

A. Incidence: up to 15% in reproductive age women, doubles in infertile women.

B. Risk Factors:
1. Nulliparous
2. age 25-40
3. infertility
4. first degree relative with endometriosis
5. improved with prior pregnancy

C. Etiologic Theories
1. retrograde menstruation
2. vascular/lymphatic dissemination
3. coelomic metaplasia
4. immunologic defect
5. genetic predisposition

D. Sites of Implants
1. Ovaries
2. Uterosacrals/posterior cul-de-sac
3. round and broad ligaments, tubes
4. rectosigmoid
5. bladder
6. extraperitoneal - cervix, vagina, vulva, incisions, umbilicus, lung. Also lymph node involvement.

E. Appearance:
1. Gross - may be new blood-filled lesions appearing red or blue/black, appearing raised or cystic. With time become flatter and dark brown. Large cystic structures may remain filled with old blood and are called chocolate cysts. Old lesions may appear as pale scarred areas puckering local tissue. Sized can range from small 1 mm lesions to cysts>10cm.
2. Histologic -
   a. ectopic endometrial glands
   b. ectopic endometrial stroma
   c. hemorrhage into adjacent tissue

F. Symptoms:
1. pelvic pain, especially secondary dysmenorrhea
2. infertility
3. dysparunia
4. abnormal uterine bleeding
5. rectal or urinary pain/bleeding associated with menses

G.   Signs:
1. fixed retroverted uterus
2. nodularity of uterosacrals and posterior cul-de-sac
3. adnexal masses, usually not symmetrical
4. tenderness on bimanual exam
5. visible lesions on speculum or external exam

H.   Diagnostic evaluation: Visualization of endometriosis is required to make diagnosis.
1. pelvic ultrasound - evaluate masses
2. laparoscopy - visualize and biopsy lesions
3. biopsy of external or vaginal lesions
4. CA-125 becomes elevated so may prove useful in follow-up

I.   Complications:
1. Adhesions - may involve genitourinary structures or bowel rupture of cysts
2. Infertility

J.   Hormonal Influence evident because:
1. rare before menarche
2. resolves after menopause
3. stabilizes or improves during pregnancy
4. incidence decreased by early and frequent pregnancies

K.   Treatment: Depends on patient's reproductive plans
1. Hormonal
   a. Oral contraceptives - taken continuously to produce months of amenorrhea (pseudopregnancy)
   b. GnRH analogues - suppresses ovarian-pituitary axis and lowers levels of FSH, LH, and estrogen creating pseudo menopause
   c. Progesterone (medroxyprogesterone)
   d. Danazol - androgen creating pseudo menopause
2. Surgical
   a. Palliative - laparoscopy or laparotomy to remove cysts, lyse adhesions, laser implants.
   b. Definitive - hysterectomy, possible oophorectomy, rarely partial colectomy with colostomy for GI involvement.

American Fertility Society Classification of Endometriosis

Patient's name _____

Stage I   (Mild)   1–5
Stage II   (Moderate)   6–15
Stage III (Severe)   16–30
Stage IV   (Extensive)   31–54

Total _____

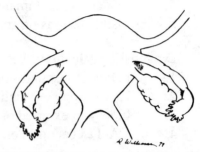

	ENDOMETRIOSIS		<1 cm	1–3 cm	> 3 cm
PERITONEUM			1	2	3
	ADHESIONS		filmy	dense w/ partial cul-de-sac obliteration	dense w/ complete cul-de-sac obliteration
			1	2	3
OVARY	ENDOMETRIOSIS		<1 cm	1–3 cm	> 3 cm or ruptured endometrioma
		R	2	4	6
		L	2	4	6
	ADHESIONS		filmy	dense w/ partial ovarian enclosure	dense w/ complete ovarian enclosure
		R	2	4	6
		L	2	4	6
TUBE	ENDOMETRIOSIS		<1 cm	> 1 cm	tubal occlusion
		R	2	4	6
		L	2	4	6
	ADHESIONS		filmy	dense w/ tubal distortion	dense w/ tubal enclosure
		R	2	4	6
		L	2	4	6

Associated Pathology:

American Fertility Society classification of endometriosis. (From the American Fertility Society: Classification of endometriosis. Fertil Steril 32:633, 1979. Reproduced with the permission of the publisher, The American Fertility Society, Birmingham, Alabama)

ADENOMYOSIS

I. **Definition** - The presence of endometrial glands and stroma within the myometrium of the uterus.

 A. Incidence - May be up to 60% but varies depending on age.

 B. Pathology -
 1. Gross - enlargement of uterus, either globally or focally. Spongy appearance, no cleavage plane,
 2. Histologically - direct extension of basalis layer of endometrium into myometrium. Rarely responsive to cyclic hormones. May:
 a. Uniformly involved uterus
 b. Focal areas that may have pseudo capsule.

 C. Symptoms:
 1. Secondary dysmenorrhea
 2. Menorrhagia
 3. Dysparunia
 4. Asymptomatic

 D. Signs: Enlarged uterus, 2-3 times normal, tender uterus, especially perimenstrually

 E. Diagnostic tests: Endometrial biopsy to rule out pathology for menorrhagia; ultrasound - may help evaluate for leiomyoma
 Confirmed By Histologic Evaluation Of Hysterectomy Specimen

 F. Treatment: trials of cyclic hormones, of prostaglandin synthetase inhibitors

Definitive Treatment By Hysterectomy

CHRONIC PELVIC PAIN

I. **Definition:** Present for > 6 months and interferes with daily functions and relationships

II. **History**

    A. Pain
        1. Duration, character, location, exacerbating or relieving factors, associated discomforts, severity, pain pattern, worsening/improving, incapacitating?

    B. Past
        1. prior infections, treatments, surgeries, diagnostic procedures, diagnoses, other medical problems, menstrual history

    C. Psychological
        1. prior diagnosis, treatments

    D. Social
        1. family dynamics, financial status, job/job stress, children, spousal relationship, recent life or lifestyle changes, sleep and diet changes

    E. Sexual
        1. association with pain, orgasmic, prior counseling or therapy, abuse or incest, inhibited desire, frequency of intercourse

III. **Examination**

    A. General physical with abdominal exam

    B. Pelvic to include evaluation for externally causes of superficial dyspareunia, lubrication; evidence of pelvic relation; masses or tenderness of adnexa, uterus or parametria; mobility, position, size of uterus; evidence of infection such as discharge, GC, chlamydia, and erobic

    C. Pap smear, stool guaiac

    D. Laboratory work - CBC, US with culture, BhCG if indicated by history, VDRL, Sedimentation rate, cervical cultures

IV. **Possible Etiologies**

    A. Gynecologic
        1. Pelvic Inflammatory Disease
        2. Pelvic Adhesions
        3. Endometriosis
        4. Pelvic Relaxation
        5. Dysmenorrhea

6.   Adenomyosis
7.   Chronic ectopic
8.   Ovarian cystic growth or bleeding
9.   Leiomyoma

B.   Urinary
1.   Bladder infection, spasm, caliculi, tumor

C.   Gastrointestinal
1.   Constipation
2.   Irritable Bowel Syndrome
3.   Inflammatory problems
4.   Appendicitis
5.   Diverticulitis
6.   Ulcerative colitis

D.   Psychological
1.   Depression
2.   Obese
3.   Stress
4.   Somatization

E.   Musculoskeletal/Neurologic
1.   Pudendal neuralgia
2.   Myofascial

V.   Diagnostic Procedures

A.   Sonogram
1.   Evaluate for masses

B.   Hysterosalpingogram
1.   can demonstrate hydrosalpinx, tubal occlusions

C.   Hysteroscopy
1.   evaluate for polyps, leiomyoma

D.   Laparoscopy
1.   can evaluate for pelvic pathology
2.   may provide tubal patency information as an HSG would
3.   will allow for treatment attempts by laser or cautery for endometriosis
4.   lysis of adhesions
5.   aspiration of cysts
6.   uterosacral ablation
7.   myomectomy
8.   oophorectomy

VI. **Studies For Non-Gynecologic Etiologies**

    A.   Psychiatric
        1.   evaluation for depression
        2.   abuse history

    B.   GI
        1.   colonoscopy or BE for lower GI tract (i.e. colitis)

    C.   Urology
        1.   cystoscope for urethritis
        2.   urolithiasis

    D.   Musculoskeletal
        1.   posture related
        2.   myofascial syndrome

VII. **Treatment**

    A.   Perform studies as indicated by history and examination

    B.   Have the patient keep a diary of pain and associated events

    C.   Medication - based on suspected etiology
        1.   NSAIDS
            a.   dysmenorrhea
            b.   mittelschmerz
            c.   uncertain?
        2.   OC's
            a.   mittelschmerz
            b.   dysmenorrhea
            c.   Not Narcotics
        3.   Tricyclics antidepressants
            a.   psychosomatic
        4.   Laparoscopy
            a.   tubal insufflation
            b.   adhesiolysis
            c   ablation of lesions - laser as indicated by findings
            d.   if normal pelvis, continue non-steroidals and counseling
            e.   if pathology is found, be prepared for TAH/BSO
        5.   Counseling as indicated for family dynamics
            a.   sexual therapy
            b.   depression
            c.   stress management
            d.   group therapy, etc.
        6.   If all therapy fails, a TAH/BSO may be performed. The possible lack of cure may be 50% if no pathology is found

REPRODUCTIVE ENDOCRINOLOGY

SEXUAL DIFFERENTIATION

Female	Embryologic Structure	Male
Ovary	Genital ridge (undifferentiated gonad)	testis
Ovarian ligament Round ligament	gubernaculum	gubernaculum testis
epoophoron paroophoron	mesonephric ridge (tubules)	epididymis paradidymis
Gartners duct Appendix of ovary	mesonephric duct	ductus deferens seminal vesicles appendix of epididymis
renal collecting system	metanephric duct	renal collecting system
fallopian tube uterus upper vagina hydatid cyst of Morgagni	paramesonephric duct (Mullerian duct)	prostatic utricle appendix of testis

lower vagina
vaginal vestibule
urinary bladder
urethra
urethral and
  paraurethral glands
greater vestibular
  glands
hymen
	urogenital sinus	urinary bladder
		prostate
		prostatic utricle
		bulbourethral glands
		urethra (non glandular)
		seminal collicle

clitoris corpora cavernosa clitoridis bulb of vestibule	genital tubercle	glans of penis corpora cavernosa and spongiosum of penis
labia minora vestibular bulbs	urethral plate	cavernous urethra
labia minora	urogenital folds	ventral portion of penis
labia majora	labioscrotal swellings	scrotum

MENSTRUAL PHYSIOLOGY

I. Divisions of the Human Menstrual Cycle

A. The Follicular Phase

1. Follows menstruation

2. There is an increase in Follicular Stimulating Hormone (FSH) which stimulates the growth and maturation of follicles

3. There is a transition from a slow to a high LH pulse frequency

4. The synthesis and release of LH and FSH are regulated by GnRH (LHRH), which is synthesized in neurons in the hypothalamus, released into the hypophysial portal vessels and transported via axoplasmic flow to the anterior pituitary gland

5. There is a recruitment of follicles during the first 4 to 5 days of the follicular phase

6. On days 5 to 7 there is a selection of a dominant follicle. The remaining follicles in the cohort may undergo additional limited growth but will ultimately become atretic

7. Maturation of a dominant follicle occurs between days 8 and 12

8. The dominant follicle reaches a mean diameter of a 20 mm several days before the LH surge

9. Theca cells have LH receptors and respond to LH stimulation by the production of androgens, primarily androstenedione and testosterone

10. Granulosa cells, which are located inside the follicle, are primarily concerned with the production of estrogens.

B. Ovulatory Phase

1. Ovulation most often occurs between days 13 and 15

2. The phase begins 2 to 3 days prior to the mid-cycle surge of Luteinizing Hormone (LH)

3. There is an increase in 17β estradiol which parallels small increases in progesterone;
17α-OH progesterone and inhibin also increase

4. The increase in progesterone reflects the process of luteinization of granulosa cells following acquisition of LH receptors and the resulting ability of LH to initiate biosynthesis of progesterone and 17α-OH progesterone

5. LH and FSH surges begin abruptly and are temporally associated with peak estradiol 17β levels and the initiation of a rapid rise in progesterone 12 hr earlier

6. The duration of the LH surge is in the range of 48 hr

7. Ovulation occurs about 36 hr after the onset of the LH surge

C. Luteal Phase
1. Following ovulation, there is a luteinization (the conversion of granulosa and theca cells to luteal cells with the acquisition of LH receptors). After this occurs luteal cells can synthesize and secrete large amounts of progesterone and to a less extent, estrogens

2. In women, following ovulation, there is an increase in the basal body temperature by 0.5 to 1.0 degree F. This is because the progesterone metabolite, pregnanediol, has a thermogenic effect and alters the setting of the thermoregulatory center in the brain

3. At the time of peak progesterone secretion, there is a 3 day window during which the endometrium is most conducive to implantation

4. Unless implantation is initiated, luteolysis (death of the corpus luteum) occurs

5. The corpus luteum needs appropriate LH (or hCG, if pregnancy is established) support to continue the secretion of progesterone

6. Levels of FSH are lowest during the luteal phase, which is due to the combined actions of inhibin, and estrogen (acting synergistically with progesterone). This prevents the initiation of folliculogenesis

D. Menstrual Phase
1. As progesterone and inhibit levels fall, there is a rise in FSH levels, which occurs 2 days prior to the onset of menses

2. This is the time at which follicular recruitment for the ensuing is initiated

3. The process of menstruation is due to declining levels of progesterone and to a lesser extent, estrogen

II. Uterine Changes During the Menstrual Cycle

A. The uterus is composed of two basic layers; the outer thick myometrium and the inner, thin, glandular tissue, the endometrium

B. The endometrium responds to estrogen, which is produced by developing follicles and undergoes rapid mitotic divisions and formation of glandular structures (proliferative endometrium)

C. After ovulation, the corpus luteum is producing significant amounts of progesterone which acts on the endometrium to increase the size of the endometrial glands and to promote the synthesis and secretion of proteins and other factors (secretory endometrium) in preparation for pregnancy and implantation

D. The secretory endometrium is maintained by the secretion of estrogen and progesterone by the ovary

E.	The decrease in the peripheral levels of these steroids causes degeneration and necrosis of the secretory endometrium and menses occurs

## III.	Cervical Changes During the Menstrual Cycle

A.	In the follicular phase there is secretion of cervical mucus by the sebaceous glands in the endocervix which is directly due to the effect of estrogen

B.	During estrogen dominance there is an abundant secretion of cervical mucus which has a characteristic "watery" appearance

C.	The elasticity of the cervical mucus is directly dependent upon the presence of estrogen and the absence of progesterone

D.	The measurement of elasticity is referred to as the "Spinnbarkeit"

E.	Also, under estrogen dominance, cervical mucus contains a large amount of NaCl and when a sample of mucus is dried it leaves a distinct "ferning pattern"

F.	When progesterone becomes the dominant hormone the cervical mucus becomes thick and the ferning pattern disappears

G.	Under progesterone dominance sperm penetration of the cervical mucus is inhibited (hostile mucus)

## IV.	Vaginal Changes During the Menstrual Cycle

A.	With a high estrogen background there is a large amount of glycogen stored in the vaginal epithelium

B.	There is a substantial change in vaginal exfoliative cytology as a result of stage of the menstrual cycle, which is a reflection of changing hormone patterns

## V.	The Process of Menstruation

A.	Menstruation
1.	Is always preceded by vasoconstriction of the spiral arteries at the base of the endometrium
2.	This results in endometrial necrosis and damage to the endothelium of the endometrial blood vessels so that when the arterioles relax, hemorrhage ensues
3.	It is now known that this hemorrhaging is due to the release of several local vasodilators including histamine, bradykinin, prostacyclin and other prostaglandins

PUBERTY

I. **Definition:** Transition from childhood to adulthood involving physiological and psychological changes

II. **Sequence of Events**   **Average Age**

    A.   Thelarche: onset of breast development   10.5 yrs.

    B.   Adrenarche: growth of pubic and axillary hair   11.0 yrs

    C.   Growth spurt: accelerated growth   11.5 yrs

    D.   Menarche: onset of menstrual period   12.8 yrs

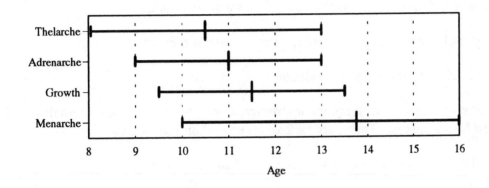

III. **Hormonal Events**

    A.   Estrogen, FSH, LH are low prior to puberty

    B.   FSH rises first, then LH, then estrogen

    C.   Pulses of LH appear, first during sleep

    D.   Estrogen increases causing changes in breast, bones, uterus and vagina

    E.   Adrenal androgens increase causing pubic and axillary hair growth

    F.   Menarche occurs when the CNS-pituitary-gonadal feedback loop is fully established

Hypothalamic-Pituitary-Gonadal Axis

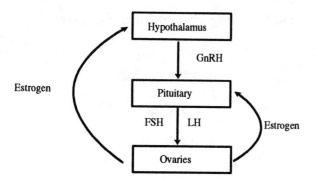

IV. Pubertal Facts

A.   Average length of puberty is four years. 1.5-8 is a normal range

B.   Ovulatory cycles are usually established after 2 years of menses

C.   Adrenal contributes to androgen production

D.   Males show pubertal development approximately 1 year later than females and are controlled by androgens. They may be 2 years behind on growth spurt.

E.   Breast and pubic hair changes are staged by the Tanner system

V. Abnormalities of Puberty

A.   Precocious puberty: onset of pubertal events (secondary sexual development) prior to age 8 in girls and age 9 in boys. This is more than 2.5 SD below the mean
   1.   Types
      a.   Isosexual: precocity appropriate for genetic and gonadal sex. Most common type
      b.   True-premature activation of hypothalamic-pituitary-gonadal axis with GnRH pulses. Causes include idiopathic (90%), CNS tumors, infections or injuries
      c.   Pseudo-not dependent on GnRH but from gonads or adrenals. Causes include estrogen producing ovarian cysts or tumor, adrenal tumors, hypothyroidism, McCune-Albright syndrome, estrogen containing medications
      d.   Heterosexual: inappropriate for genetic sex. Includes feminizing of males or virilizing of females. Most common etiology is CAH or androgen producing adrenal or ovarian tumors
   2.   Etiologies
      a.   Idiopathic
      b.   Ovarian cyst or tumor
      c.   Central nervous system disorder or tumor

        d.   McCune-Albright syndrome
        e.   Adrenal tumor or hyperplasia
        f.   Ectopic gonadotropin production
        g.   Hypothyroidism
        h.   Exogenous estrogen consumption

3.   Diagnostic tests
        a.   LH
        b.   FSH
        c.   GnRH stimulation
        d.   Estradiol
        e.   Testosterone
        f.   DHEAS
        g.   Prolactin
        h.   Thyroid function
        i.   17-OHP
        j.   Radiologic tests to rule out CNS
        k.   Gonadal and adrenal tumor
        l.   History and physical exam always included. Bone age determination

4.   Treatment
        a.   Surgery as indicated for tumors
        b.   GnRH analogue for idiopathic/constitutional (Lupron, Synarel)

B.   Delayed puberty: absence of thelarche by age 13 or menarche by age 15. Occurs < 1% of the time

1.   Types
        a.   Constitutional delay: most common showing delay of onset of GnRH pulse generator. Once puberty begins events are normal.
        b.   Hypogonadotropic hypogonadism - GnRH, FSH or LH deficiency etiologies include CNS tumors or infections, isolated gonadotropin deficiency, functional (anorexia), and other syndromes.
        c.   Hypergonadotropic hypogonadism: gonadal failure with elevated FSH and LH and decreased estrogen. Etiologies include Turner's syndrome in the female and Klinefelter's in males

2.   Diagnostic tests
        a.   H & P
        b.   Growth chart bone age determination
        c.   Karyotype
        d.   LH
        e.   FSH
        f.   GnRH stimulation test
        g.   evaluation for tumors

3.   Treatment - based on etiology
        a.   May be expectant or involve hormonal therapy
        b.   Females need estrogen and progestins and males need testosterone
        c.   Include counseling as needed for psychological issues

ABNORMAL UTERINE BLEEDING

I. **Introduction**

    A.   Limits of Normal
        1.   Cycle 21-35 days
        2.   Lasts 2-7 days
        3.   Not over eight soaked pads/day, usually not over two heavy daysAnemia, observe patient bleeding
        4.   Changes are important.

    B.   Definitions
        1.   Hypermenorrhea - too much bleeding, also referred to as Menorrhagia. Normal cycles.
        2.   Polymenorrhea - too much frequent or irregular bleeding; also - Metrorrhagia.

    C.   Physiology
        1.   Ovulation synchronizes spiral arteriolar spasm. Subsequent ischemia, necrosis, and regular endometrial shedding.

II. **Organic Etiology**

    A.   Reproductive Tract Disease
        1.   Pregnancy complications - most common:
            Abortion
            Ectopic Occasionally

        2.   Intrauterine benign neoplasia - polyp, myoma

        3.   Reproductive tract malignancy

        4.   Cervicitis, endometritis, salpingitis

        5.   Endometriosis

        6.   Adenomyosis

        7.   Functional cysts

        8.   IUD

    B.   Systemic Disease
        1.   Blood Dyscrasias - Thrombocytopenia
        2.   Hypo or hyperthyroidism
        3.   Liver disease
        4.   Obesity
        5.   Diabetes
        6.   Hypertension
        7.   Adrenal Disorders

III. Dysfunctional Etiology

    A.   Term used after organic and iatrogenic causes ruled out.

    B.   Predominantly result of anovulation, so etiology hormonal

    C.   10 - 15% cases of dysfunctional uterine bleeding associated with ovulatory cycles.

    D.   If patient ovulates, cause of bleeding is usually mechanical, (fibroids, etc.) and hormonal therapy unlikely to be helpful. Thus, sampling of endometrium in second half of cycle will help establish diagnosis and prognosis.

IV. Diagnosis

    A.   Careful history

    B.   Physical exam

    C.   Rule out pregnancy, thyroid disease, blood dyscrasias, etc.

    D.   Pelvic exam whether bleeding or not
        1.   Pap smear
        2.   Sounding of uterus
        3.   Endometrial sampling, pipette, etc., in second half of cycle

    E.   Hysteroscopy or HSG - if normal pelvic exam, ovulation documented, unresponsive to hormonal therapy.

    F.   Ultrasound

V. Treatment

Remember! Pills are not good for anything except anovulation andcontraception.

    A.   Simple observation in young adolescent with small amounts of irregular bleeding. Can use oral contraceptives, but may aggravate already suppressed hypothalamic-ovarian axis.

    B.   Sample endometrium - use local (PC block) and 2% Xylocaine gel.
        1.   Endometrial biopsy adequate to rule out cancer. Less expensive, equally sensitive to a D&C.
        2.   D&C and hysteroscopy - If you are going to go as far as an anesthetic for D&C, might as well look - Diagnostic and therapeutic - 60 - 70% cure rate with D&C alone - at least for next six months.

C.   Followed by hormonal regulation - increases cure rate to near 90% in anovulatory patients.
1.   Cyclic oral contraceptives.
2.   Cyclic progesterone injection every four weeks. Oral progesterone also appropriate.
3.   May need high dose estrogen followed by progesterone for severe bleeding.

D.   Endometrial Ablation - resection or KTP laser. Fibroids contraindicated. Adenomyoma frequently not cured.

E.   Excision of polyp or leiomyoma.

F.   Hysterectomy - only as last resort. Risk of hysterectomy about equal to risk of blood transfusion. Thus, bleeding heavy enough to cause moderate anemia that is not controlled by hormones or other therapies, warrants hysterectomy.

AMENORRHEA

I. Definition

A. **Primary Amenorrhea:** No period by age 14 in the absence of growth or development of secondary sexual characteristics or no period by age 16 regardless of the presence of normal growth and development with the appearance of secondary sexual characteristics.

B. **Secondary Amenorrhea:** In a woman who has been menstruating, the absence of periods for a length of time equivalent to a total of at least three of the previous cycle intervals, or six months of amenorrhea.

II. Possible Causes

A. Compartment I:
Disorders of outflow tract or uterine target organ

B. Compartment II:
Disorders of the Ovary

C. Compartment III:
Disorders of the Anterior Pituitary

D. Compartment IV:
Disorders of CNS (hypothalamic factors)

III. Evaluation

Step I:
Careful history - evidence for psychological dysfunction or emotional stress, family history of apparent genetic anomalies, discussion of nutritional habits, sexual activity.

Step 2:
Physical examination -
- a. Nutritional status
- b. Abnormal growth and development
- c. Evidence of CNS disease
- d. Tanner stage
- e. Evidence of other endocrine disorders (galactorrhea, enlarged thyroid)
- f. Presence of a normal reproductive tract

If Abnormality of uterus or vagina:

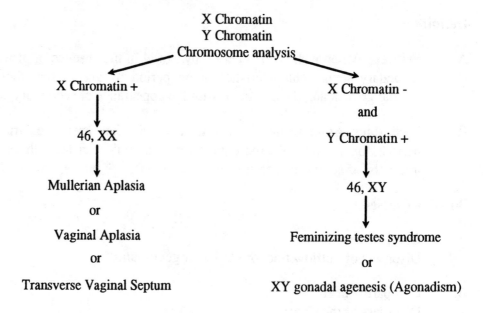

X Chromatin
Y Chromatin
Chromosome analysis

X Chromatin +

46, XX

Mullerian Aplasia

or

Vaginal Aplasia

or

Transverse Vaginal Septum

X Chromatin -

and

Y Chromatin +

46, XY

Feminizing testes syndrome

or

XY gonadal agenesis (Agonadism)

If no abnormalities, proceed to Step 3.

Step 3:
    a.   Exclude pregnancy
    b.   Measure TSH
    c.   Measure prolactin level
    d.   Perform Progestational challenge

If positive withdraw bleed, and normal prolactin/TSH diagnosis is anovulatory cycles.

If diagnosis not established and no withdraw bleeding, proceed to step 4.

Step 4.

Estrogen and Progestin Cycle - May take 2.5 mg conjugated estrogen daily for twenty-one (21) days with Provera 10 mg daily for the last five (5) days.

If withdraw bleeding does not occur, then end organ problem.

If withdraw bleeding occurs, proceed to step 5.

Step 5:

Gonadotropin Assay

If elevated and patient over the age of 30, chromosomal analysis (if mosaicism with a Y chromosome, 25% chance of malignant tumor formation).

If normal or low, proceed to step 6.

Step 6:

Coronal CT Scan - To evaluate sella turcica and suprasellar area.

IV.   Differential Diagnosis

A.   Classification of Secondary Amenorrhea
1.   Physiologic amenorrhea

2.   Iatrogenic amenorrhea

3.   End organ causes of secondary amenorrhea
   a.   Uterine adhesions
   b.   Cervical stenosis
   c.   Vesicovaginal fistula
   d.   Hormone-resistant endometrium

4.   Ovarian causes of secondary amenorrhea
   a.   Gonadal dysgenesis with limited menstrual function
   b.   Premature ovarian failure
   c.   Resistant ovaries syndrome

5.   Hypothalamic-pituitary lesions
   a.   Destructive hypothalamic-pituitary lesions
   b. Sheehan syndrome
   c.   Amenorrhea associated with increased prolactin secretion
   d.   Hypothalamic-pituitary dysfunction
   e.   Amenorrhea associated with changes in weight

6.   Psychogenic amenorrhea
   a.   Anorexia nervosa
   b.   Pseudocyesis
   c.   Amenorrhea caused by environmental changes
   d.   Secondary amenorrhea of adolescence

7.   Amenorrhea associated with thyroid disorders

8.   Amenorrhea associated with virilizing disorders
   a.   Polycystic ovaries syndrome
   b.   Ovarian hyperthecosis
   c.   Ovarian tumor
   d.   Adrenal hyperplasia
   e.   Adrenal tumor
   f.   Cushing syndrome

9.   Amenorrhea associated with systemic diseases

B.   Primary Amenorrhea
1.   Primary amenorrhea without breast development and uterus present
   a.   Gonadal failure
      1.   45, X - 50%
      2.   46, X, abnormal X (i.e., short-arm or long-arm deletion) - 25%
      3.   Mosaicism - 25%
      4.   Pure XY gonadal dysgenesis

5. XY gonadal dysgenesis - Sawyer's Syndrome
   a. XY Karyotype
   b. Palpable Mullerian system
   c. Normal female testosterone levels
   d. Lack of sexual development
6. 17-Hydroxylase deficiency (with 46, XX Karyotype)
b. CNS - hypothalamic - pituitary disorders
   1. CNS lesion
   2. Hypothalamic failure secondary to inadequate GnRH release
   3. Isolated gonadotropin insufficiency

2. Primary Amenorrhea with Breast Development and Absent Uterus
   a. Congenital absence of uterus (utero-vaginal atresia)
   b. Androgen insensitivity (testicular feminization)
      1. Normal female phenotype
      2. Normal male karyotype 46, XY
      3. Normal or slightly elevated male blood testosterone levels
      4. X-linked recessive

3. Primary Amenorrhea with no breast development and absent uterus
   a. 17, 20-Desmolase deficiency
   b. Agonadism
   c. 17-Hydroxylase deficiency (with 46, XY Karyotype)

4. Primary Amenorrhea with Breast Development and Uterus Present
   a. Hypothalamic causes
   b. Pituitary causes
   c. Ovarian causes
   d. Uterine causes

HIRSUTISM AND VIRILISM

I. **Definitions**

   A. Hirsutism - Presence of excessive facial and body hair. May be present as a normal variant or may be due to excessive androgen production in a female.

   B. Virilism - Presence of mature masculine somatic characteristics in a female. May be present at birth or develop later in life. Results from excessive androgen.

II. **Biology of Hair Growth**

   A. Follicles develop at 8 weeks gestation

   B. Distribution varies with ethnicity but does not vary by sex

   C. Lanugo growth occurs in utero

   D. Sexual hair responds to sex steroids

   E. Sexual hair grows on face, lower abdomen, anterior thighs, chest, pubic area, axilla

   F. Androgens initiate sexual hair growth
       1. Testosterone is major circulating androgen
       2. Dihydrotestosterone (DHT) is major nuclear androgen at follicle
       3. 3a-Androstanediol is peripheral tissue metabolite of DHT
       4. 3a-Androstanediol glucuronide is utilized as marker of tissue action

   G. Estrogens retard sexual hair growth

   H. Progestins have minimal effect on hair growth

   I. Hair growth phases
       1. Anagen - growing phase
       2. Catagen - rapid involution phase
       3. Telogen - quiescent phase

III. **Biology of Virilism**

   A. Androgens act on testosterone receptive tissues

   B. Breast - atrophy

   C. Striated muscle - hypertrophy

   D. Clitoromegaly

   E. Endometrial and uterine atrophy

   F. Vocal cord coarsening and deepening of voice

IV. Sources of Androgen

    A.   Excess androgen comes from one of three sources - ovarian, adrenal or exogenous. Normally 50 % of circulating testosterone comes from peripheral conversion of androstenedione, with 25 % from ovary and 25 % from adrenal

    B.   Ovarian
        1.   Androstenedione production is increased with polycystic ovary syndrome

        2.   Dehydroepiandrosterone (DHA) my be produced by ovary

        3.   With excessive stromal tissue, testosterone becomes significant secretory product

        4.   Androgenic tumors
            a.   Sertoli- Leydig cell tumors (arrhenoblastomas)
            b.   Hilus cell tumors
            c.   Lipoid cell (adrenal rest) tumors
            d.   Rarely granulosa-thecal cell tumors

    C.   Adrenal
        1.   Dehydroepiandrosterone sulfate (DHAS) is almost exclusively of adrenal origin
        2.   90 % of DHA comes from adrenal
        3.   Cushing's syndrome
        4.   Adult congenital adrenal hyperplasia - incomplete 21 hydroxylase or 11B hydroxylase deficiency

    D.   Exogenous
        1.   Testosterone is often given to women in combination with estrogens by injection or oral forms - depo testosterone may have androgenic effects for long periods of time
        2.   Anabolic steroids may be used illicitly for body building
        3.   Danocrine sulfate used for endometriosis

V. Evaluation of Hirsutism/Virilism

    A.   Physical examination
        1.   Ovarian size
        2.   Signs of Cushing's

    B.   Laboratory evaluation
        1.   Serum testosterone - normal 20 - 80 ng/dl
        2.   DHAS - Normal < 700 ug/dl
        3.   17-hydroxyprogesterone - Normals - 15 - 70 ng/dl follicular, 35 - 290 ng/dl luteal

4.   Flow diagram of workup

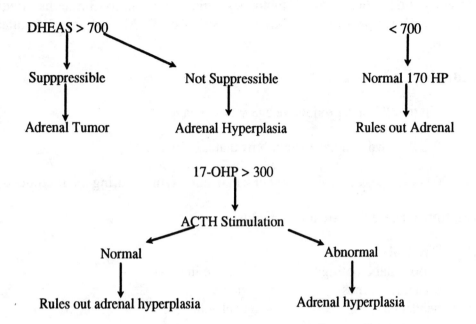

Serum T, DHEAS, 17-OHP normal ⟶ Idiopathic hirsutism

Serum T > 200 ⟶ Suspect androgen producing tumor

DHEAS > 700   < 700

Suppressible   Not Suppressible   Normal 170 HP

Adrenal Tumor   Adrenal Hyperplasia   Rules out Adrenal

17-OHP > 300

ACTH Stimulation

Normal   Abnormal

Rules out adrenal hyperplasia   Adrenal hyperplasia

VI.   Therapy

A   Directed toward reduction of androgen

B.   Specific therapy depends on source of androgen
1.   Ovarian
a.   Suppression of LH - Oral contraceptive pills
b.   If OCP contraindicated, medroxyprogesterone acetate
c.   In older woman resistant to hormone therapy, consider oophorectomy
d.   If functioning ovarian tumor found, surgical removal

2.   Adrenal
a.   Glucocorticoid replacement
b.   Surgical removal of tumors

PREMENSTRUAL SYNDROME

I.   **Definition -** a group of symptoms that occur during the luteal phase of the menstrual cycle. The are relieved with the onset of menses or within 2-3 days of menses. There should be a symptom free period of time during the follicular phase of at least one week. Symptoms often interfere with work and relationships. Symptoms should be present for 3 months. Requires the woman to ovulatory. A severe form of PMS is classified by DSM - III as a late luteal phase dysphoric disorder.

II. **Incidence:**

   A.   Up to 40% of reproductive age women have PMS.

   B.   2-3% of women have symptoms that are severe.

III. **Age:** 30's-40's (peaking mid 30's) but can occur anytime during the reproductive years.

IV. **Symptoms:** These lists are not all inclusive

   A.   Physical
abdominal bloating	change in bowels
breast tendernes	sacne
headache	backache
leg cramps/swelling	crave sweets/salt
pelvic pain	palpitations
incoordination	sensitivity to noise/light
increased appetite	rash/itching
nasal congestion	hot flush

   B.   Emotional
depression	hostility
anxiety	anger
inability to cope	paranoia
fatigue	change in sex drive
tearfulness	poor concentration
aggression/violence	insecurity
forgetfulness	suicidal thoughts
insomnia	desire to be alone
tension	guilt feelings
irritability	weakness

V. Pathophysiological Theories:

A. increased estrogen

B. decreased B6

C. elevated prolactin

D. hypoglycemia

E. fluid retention

F. prostaglandin abnormalities

G. endorphin withdrawal

H. hypothyroidism

I. increased MAO

J. hormone allergy

VI. Evaluation Methods:

A. Patient history

B. Examination for organic pathology, because there are NO objective physical findings for PMS

C. Symptom diary best - should keep for 2-3 months to look for a clustering of symptoms.

D. Basal body temperature chart to document ovulation.

E. Menstrual calendar - usually part of BBT.

F. Personality/Psychological testing - ex.MMMPI, Beck depression inventory, Hamilton Depression scale, Zung's anxiety scale, etc. Need to differentiate from depression.

G. Labs - TSH, prolactin, fasting blood sugar

VII. Treatment Methods:

A. Education to understand premenstrual syndrome.

B. Nutrition - small meals high in protein, vitamins and complex carbohydrates. Low in fat and no refined sugars. Alcohol, tobacco and caffeine are to be avoided. Salt is limited. Vitamin B 6 may be added.

C. Exercise - 30 minutes of daily aerobics; may increase endorphins.

D.   Stress management

E.   Counseling/psychotherapy to supplement other treatment. This may be individual or include support groups.

F.   Hormone therapy - natural progesterone is no more effective than placebo. Medroxyprogesterone acetate, oral contraceptives, GnRH agonists, given to stop menstruation..

G.   Other medical therapy aimed at specific symptomatology -
       1.   Diuretics (potassium sparing)
       2.   Antidepressants
       3.   Anxiolytics
       4.   Anti prostaglandins (NSAIDS)
       5.   Bromocriptine (for breast tenderness)
       6.   Vitamin B6 (cofactor for serotonin)
       7.   Clonidine
       8.   Antiprostaglandins for breast tenderness, joint pain, musculoskeletal pain.

INFERTILITY

I.   **Definition:** one year of unprotected intercourse without pregnancy.

II.   **Incidence:** 10% of population

III.   **Fertility rate:** 20% per cycle; number of births/1000 women age 15-44

IV.   **Physiology of Reproduction:**

    A.   Fimbria: bring ova into tube, while about 200 million sperm are deposited in the vagina.

    B.   Estimated life-span: sperm - 48 hours; ova - 12-24 hours

    C.   Capacitation of sperm occurs

    D.   Fertilization occurs in ampulla of tube, ova completes meiosis II and extrudes 2nd polar body

    E.   Implantation occurs day 6-7 after ovulation

V.   **Causes of Infertility**

    A.   Tubal disease - 25-50%

    B.   Anovulation - 20-40%

    C.   Male factor - 40%

    D.   Cervical factor - 5-10%

    E.   Unknown - 10%

    F.   Peritoneal factor - 5-10%

    G.   Uterine/endometrial i.e. luteal phase defect - 3-10%

    H.   Combination

VI.   **Evaluation**

    A.   History
        1.   Pubertal events
        2   Menstrual History - amenorrhea, oligo-ovulation etc.
        3.   Abnormal hair growth, galactorrhea, dyspareunia, pelvic pain, pelvic infections, acne, visual symptoms, headaches.
        4.   Previous contraception, especially IUD
        5.   Frequency of coitus

6. Duration of pregnancy attempts.
7. History of genital trauma or infection in husband, mumps after puberty.
8. DES exposure
9. Current medications
10. Partner's history - prior children, illnesses

B. Physical Exam - Routine speculum and bimanual pelvic exam

C. Semen analysis - should be $\geq$ 20 million/cc, $\geq$ 60% motile and $\geq$ 60% normal morphology. Normal volume 3-5 cc. Abstain 48-72 prior to giving specimen. Follow up in 2-3 months if repeat needed.

D. Basal body temperature chart (BBT) - Temperature should go up 1° F 24 hours after ovulation. Coincides with rise in progesterone levels to >4 ng/ml. A biphasic curve confirms ovulation, however some ovulatory women may have monophasic curve.

E. Postcoital test - Performed on expected day of ovulation. Observe 48 hours of sexual abstinence, then have intercourse. The cervical mucus is examined within 8 hours of intercourse. The following things are evaluated:
1. Quality of mucus - thick vs. thin, opaque vs. clear
2. Spinnbarkeit - should be 8-10 cm
3. Presence of ferning
4. Sperm/hpf - motility, direction, morphology, 1-20/hpf

F. Hysterosalpingogram - to evaluate tubal patency and contour of uterine cavity. Should be performed day 10 of cycle. Contraindicated in presence of pelvic infection.

G. Endometrial biopsy - Should be performed 2-3 days before expected menses (day 26). Can be used to confirm ovulation (secretory endometrium), but main purpose is to look for luteal phase defect.

H. Laparoscopy - if all the above tests are normal, laparoscopy may be used to evaluate unsuspected anatomic factors; can also be used earlier in the workup if endometriosis is suspected or a past history of pelvic pathology.

VII. Treatment

A. Tubal Factors - non-patent tubes are frequently due to PID.
1. 1st episode PID - 10-15% infertility.
2. 2nd episode PID - 25% infertility.
3. 3rd episode PID - 50% infertility.
    Lysis of tubal adhesions and tubal reconstruction may restore tubal patency.
    Tubal patency, however does not guarantee successful pregnancy.

B. Anovulation or Oligo- ovulation - very common cause of infertility. Must rule out underlying endocrine disorders prior to therapy.

Hormonal assays - TSH, prolactin, DHEA-sulfate. If premature ovarian failure or hypothalamic amenorrhea is suspected an FSH and LH will also help.

Women who are morbidly obese or very thin (anorexia nervosa, ballet dancer, runners, etc) will frequently be anovulatory. Restoration of ideal body weight is usually needed to restore ovulation.

Tests for ovulation:
1. BBT
2. Endometrial bx showing secretory endometrium
3. Serum progesterone greater than 4ng/ml on day 21
4. Dysmenorrhea and premenstrual Sx's are very unusual in women who are not ovulating.
5. Regular, cyclical, predictable menses suggests ovulatory cycles.
6. Detection of LH surge in urine

Therapy for anovulation - correct the underlying endocrine abnormality, if there is one. If not, ovulation induction is indicated (clomiphene or Pergonal).

C. Cervical Factor - Poor cervical mucus can be a barrier to sperm penetration. Low dose estrogen on days 5-13 during mid-follicular phase may improve the mucus. Artificial insemination of washed sperm into uterine cavity can be used to bypass cervical mucus. Donor mucus also a possibility.

D. Male Factors:
1. Infection - especially prostate, epididymis
2. Mumps as an adult
3. Testicular injury, torsed testicle, etc.
4. Varicocele
5. Heat - increased scrotal temperature can decrease sperm count and motility.
6. Drugs - marijuana use may decrease sperm count; chemotherapy
7. Smoking - can decrease motility, count and morphology.
8. Alcohol - can decrease testosterone. May Also decrease libido.
9. Retrograde ejaculation, hypospadias, radiation, congenital, chromosomal
10. previous vasectomy
11. sperm antibodies

Treatment:
a. Artificial insemination donor sperm (AID)
b. Artificial insemination husband sperm (AIH)
c. Correction of underlying abnormality, if possible
d. Corticosteroids may be of benefit in sperm antibodies.
e. In-vitro Fertilization (IVF).
f. Donor sperm

E.   Endometriosis - Little doubt that extensive endometriosis causing tubal and ovarian adhesions can be a cause of infertility. Less certain is the role of peritoneal endometriosis that does not involve tubes/ovaries. Many believe that even minimal endometriosis can cause infertility - ? mechanism, possibly prostaglandin mediated.

Treatment:
    a.   surgical
    b.   Birth control pills
    c.   Danocrine sulfate x 6 months
    d.   Progestins (Provera, Depo-Provera)
    e.   Long-acting GnRH agonists.

The highest pregnancy rates following conservative surgery occur in the first year after surgery.

F.   Luteal Phase Defect - Diagnosed by Endometrial biopsy. performed on day 26. Endometrium lags behind the cycle day by more than 2 days. Found in 3-4% infertile women, but 30% of all women will have an occasional luteal phase defect, therefore must show endometrial lag in 2 cycles in order to make the diagnosis. Inadequate progesterone production by corpus luteum is often the cause. Elevated prolactin can also cause.

Treatment:
    a.   Clomiphene
    b.   Progesterone supplements during luteal phase.
    c.   Bromocriptine (only if elevated prolactin).

G.   Recurrent (2 spontaneous abortions) or habitual loss (> 3 spontaneous abortions).

1.   Karyotype on male and female - 50-60% of all first trimester losses are due to some genetic defect in the conceptus.

2.   Uterine anomalies - septate uterus, T-shaped uterus (DES exposure), bicornuate uterus, etcetera. these patients typically present with a history of recurrent early 2nd Trimester losses. Also, distorting uterine leiomyomata.
*Remember - always look for associated renal anomalies.
Treatment - some can be surgically corrected.

3.   Intrauterine adhesions (Asherman's Syndrome) - typically present with secondary infertility and/or amenorrhea or oligo-menorrhea. Classically follows a pregnancy-related D&C. Treatment is resection of adhesions through the hysteroscope followed by high-dose estrogen to restore normal endometrium.

4.   Luteal phase defect - may present only as recurrent 1st trimester loss.

5.   Cervical incompetence - painless cervical dilatation with subsequent ROM and fetal loss. Usually 2nd trimester. Treatment - cerclage.

6.   Chronic infection - chlamydia, Brucella, Listeria.

7.   Metabolic/Endocrine/Chronic disease - SLE, thyroid, diabetes, adrenal, sickle cell.

8.   Immunologic - antisperm antibodies, HLA compatibility.

H.   In Vitro Fertilization
1.   GIFT (Gamete intra fallopian transfer)
2.   Donor oocytes.

MENOPAUSE

I. Definitions

A. Menopause - The cessation of menstruation. The average age in the U.S. is 51 years old with a normal range of 40-60. Due to the increasing life expectancy, approximately 1/3 of lives are spent in the post-menopausal years. May be natural, surgical or due to other influences such as XRT or chemotherapy. Occurs 2 years sooner in smokers.

B. Climacteric - The process of changing from a reproductive to a non-reproductive status. Occurs over a 3-5 year time span (perimenopause).

II. Etiology

A. Overall a problem of oocyte depletion. Peak oocyte number at 20 weeks gestation. By the 4th decade, they are more difficult to recruit to maturation, leading to anovulation and irregular menses. Remaining follicles secrete less estrogen causing follicle stimulating hormone to rise.

III. Diagnosis

A. Symptoms
1. Abnormal menstrual cycles - up to 90%
2. Hot flushes (vasomotor instability) - 80%
3. Emotional lability, not depression
4. Vaginal dryness, Dysparunia
5. Bladder symptoms
6. Sleep disturbances

B. Signs
1. Vaginal and vulvar atrophy, pelvic relaxation
2. Osteoporosis
3. Cardiovascular disease
4. Altered lipid profile

C. Laboratory
1. FSH - useful in perimenopausal years if diagnosis unclear. Levels >40 mIU/ml indicate postmenopausal state
2. LH - rarely indicated. Postmenopausal if >40 mIU/ml
3. Estrogen level - usually reserved to evaluate ineffective treatment on maximum doses. Levels: 40-250 pg/ml = normal; <20 pg/ml = menopausal
4. Vaginal maturation index - a smear of vaginal mucosa to evaluate the percentage of basal, parabasal, and superficial cells present. An estrogen dominant environment will have a majority of superficial cells

IV.   Complications

A.   Osteoporosis - Most common fracture site vertebrae, then femur and forearm. Over 1 million fractures/year with 2/3 of them in women. Maximum bone density achieved in early 30's. Height loss of 2.5 inches during lifetime. Vertebral facture in 1/3 of women over 65. Estrogen + calcium exercise is the best prevention. Hip fracture occurs in 1/3 of women over 90 with a 10-15% mortality rate. Risk factors include caucasian, thin, short stature, sedentary, family history, smoking, steroid use, hyperthyroidism, blood thinning medications, caffeine, alcohol and any reason for decreased estrogen and other medical illness. Estrogen decreases bone resorption and improves calcium absorption. Progestins added actually increase bone formation.

B.   Cardiovascular disease - #1 cause of death in postmenopausal women. Estrogen replacement therapy decreased risk by 50% with improvement for current users > those who were never users. Increase in total cholesterol and low density lipoproteins occurs

C.   Psychosexual changes - most likely related to changes in the genital tissue causing discomfort with intercourse

D.   Endometrial cancer - a risk if estrogen taken unopposed by progesterone in a women with a uterus. Combination of estrogen and progesterone actually decreases risk more than no hormonal therapy. Can follow stimulation to endometrium with endometrial biopsies or ultrasound measurement of endometrial thickness (biopsy if > 5 mm).

E.   Gallbladder disease - 1.5-2 times the relative risk

F.   Breast cancer - inconclusive data but felt to be related to increased estrogen exposure throughout life (early menarche, late menopause, delayed childbearing) or exogenous estrogen exposure of 15 years or greater

V.   Treatment

A.   Estrogen - lowers LDL's and raises HDL's, lowers total cholesterol. Begin in first 3 years of menopause. Adequate daily doses include 0.625 mg conjugated equine estrogen, 1.0 mg micronized estradiol, and 0.05 mg transdermal 17β estradiol and 5-10ug ethinyl estradiol. Regimens vary. Cyclic therapy with > 50% withdraw bleeds and continuous methods with 5% bleeding after 1 year of therapy and 35% only during first 6 months. FDA-approved for treatment of osteoporosis. Increases calcitonin

B.   Calcium - 1000 mg/day if on estrogen and 1500 mg/day if not of elemental calcium. Calcium carbonate best.

C.   Exercise - weight bearing

D.   Progesterone - may help hot flushes and osteoporosis. Formulations include medroxyprogesterone acetate (Provera), micronized progesterone, and norethindrone. If used daily, doses include 2.5-5 mg, 200 mg and .35 mg, respectively.

E. Calcitonin - prevents bone resorption. FDA-approved as a treatment for osteoporosis. Given as an intramuscular medication

F. Oral contraceptives - during perimenopause

G. Vitamin D

H. Other medications - clonidine, etidronate

VI. Estrogen Contraindications

A. Unexplained uterine bleeding

B. Pregnancy

C. Active thrombophlebitis

D. History of thrombophlebitis associated with estrogen

E. Estrogen-dependent cancers (endometrial, breast)

GYNECOLOGIC ONCOLOGY

VULVAR NEOPLASIAS

I. Premalignant Lesions

A. Vulvar condylomata
  1. Confirm by biopsy
  2. Treatment
     a. 25-50% podophyllin
     b. 50-75% trichloroacetic acid
     c. 5% 5-fluorouracil
     d. Laser vaporization
     e. Interferon

B. Vulvar dystrophias
  1. Lichen sclerosis (LS)
     a. Confirm by biopsy
     b. Associated with autoimmune phenomena
     c. Occurs predominantly in postmenopausal women
     d. Predominant symptom is pruritus
     e. Approximately 5% of cases have an associated vulvar carcinoma at presentation.
     f. Treatment - Topical testosterone propionate 2% in white petrolatum bid/tid

  2. Hyperplastic dystrophy
     a. Represents 25 to 50% of vulvar dystrophias
     b. Patients tend to be younger than those with LS
     c. Unifocal with hyperkeratosis
     d. More often associated with dysplasia or carcinoma at diagnosis than LS
     e. Treatment - Topical Corticosteroids

  3. Mixed dystrophy
     a. Characterized by areas of both atrophic and hyperplastic dystrophy

C. Vulvar Intraepithelial Neoplasia (VIN)
  1. Etiology/Clinical features
     a. Associated with condyloma and HPV
     b. Most common symptom is pruritus
     c. May be unifocal or multifocal

  2. Evaluation
     a. Careful inspection of the entire perineum to include colposcopic evaluation
     b. Directed biopsies based upon exam
     c. Evaluate the cervix and vagina for squamous neoplasia due to relatively high risk of involvement of the entire genital tract.

3.   Treatment
    a.   Laser ablation
    b.   Skinning vulvectomy with split thickness skin graft

D.   Vulvar carcinoma
  1.   Epidemiology
    a.   Accounts for 3-5% of all female genital cancers
    b.   Average age at diagnosis is 65.
    c.   Associated conditions include hypertension, obesity and low parity
    d.   Squamous cell histology is found in approximately 87% of cases.

  2.   Symptoms
    a.   Lump, ulcer or pruritus most common clinical manifestations
    b.   Two of three women with vulvar cancer have had symptoms for greater than 6 months prior to diagnosis.

  3.   Diagnosis
    a.   Physician delay is common because vulvar cancer mimics other clinical entities. Prompt performance of office biopsy will facilitate the correct diagnosis and subsequent treatment.
    b.   A punch biopsy from the center of the lesion is the most reliable method for obtaining a pathologic diagnosis.

  4.   FIGO Stage Grouping and TNM Classification for Vulvar Carcinoma (1988)

TNM Classification			FIGO	
Designation		Description	Stage	Description
T		Primary tumor	I	T1 N0 M0
	Tis	Preinvasive carcinoma (carcinoma in situ)	II	T2 N0 M0
	T1	Tumor confined to the vulva and/or perineum, 2 cm or less in largest diameter	III	T3 N0 M0
				T3 N1 M0
				T1 N1 M0
				T2 N1 M0
	T2	Tumor confined to the vulva and/or perineum, more than 2 cm in largest diameter	IVA	T1 N2 M0
				T2 N2 M0
				T3 N2 M0
				T4 N0/N1/N2, M0
	T3	Tumor of any size with (1) adjacent spread to the lower urethra and/or vagina and/or anus and/or (2) unilateral regional lymph node metastasis	IVB	any T, any N with M1
	T4	Tumor infiltrating any of the following: upper urethra, bladder mucosa, rectal mucosa, pelvic bone and/or bilateral regional lymph node metastases		
N		Regional lymph nodes		
	N0	No node metastasis		
	N1	Unilateral node metastasis		
	N2	Bilateral node metastases		
M		Distant metastases		
	M0	No clinical metastases		
	M1	Pelvic lymph node or other distant metastases		

  5.   Treatment
    a.   Radical vulvectomy and bilateral inguinal lymph node dissection

CERVICAL NEOPLASIA

I.   **Pathophysiology of Disease**

   A.   Etiology
   1.   Epidemiologic studies have concluded that this disease follows a pattern of a sexually transmitted disease

   2.   Scientific evidence now implicates the sexually transmitted agent to be human papillomavirus
   a.   Lifetime risk of contracting virus is 1/3 or greater
   b.   Yet only 13,000 women are diagnosed with cervical cancer annually
   c.   4500 women are expected to die annually
   d.   There are other cofactors which must assist in the neoplastic process such as cigarette smoking, presence of oncogenes

   B.   Risk factors for cervix cancer
   1.   Early age of first coitus/pregnancy
   2.   Multiple sexual partners
   3.   Immune suppression
   4.   Low socioeconomic status
   5.   Lack of pap smear screening

   C.   Natural history of disease
   1.   Dysplastic process begins in the squamocolumnar junction
   a.   Progression occurs from mild dysplastic to moderate to severe dysplasia and carcinoma in situ over many years
   b.   Some patients will have more rapid transformation
   c.   Some patients may have dysplasia resolve without treatment
   d.   Average rate of development of invasive cancer is 10-20 years

   2.   Invasive cancer - defined by tumor cells breaking through the basement membrane and invading underlying stroma
   a.   Tumor then spreads by local invasion
   b.   Metastatic spread is via lymphatics to pelvic lymph nodes
   c.   Hematogenous spread is uncommon
   d.   Death usually occurs from renal failure secondary to hydronephrosis or hemorrhage from tumor site

II.   **Pap Smear - Screening Test**

   A.   Prevention of cervix cancer
   1.   Procedure to screen patients for premalignant changes

   2.   Detection of premalignant changes (dysplasia) allows for successful treatment and prevention of cancer

3. Failures of prevention
   a. Large population remains noncompliant with guidelines
      1.) Healthy women after tubal ligation
      2.) Postmenopausal women who see physicians who do not perform pelvic exams
   b. Failures of treatment of dysplasia
   c. False negative cytology report

4. Words of wisdom
   a. Pap is not a "test for cancer" it is only a screening test with a 15-40% false negative result - a negative result is no guarantee
   b. When a lesion is present - biopsy it - a pap smear should not be performed as a diagnostic test
   c. Pap smear is not a diagnostic test - it requires tissue confirmation with biopsy
   d. A pap does not adequately evaluate uterus, ovaries or tubes.

III. Diagnostic Procedures

A. Colposcopy - a technique for obtaining histologic diagnosis and treatment planning
   1. Magnified examination of cervical transformation zone - squamocolumnar junction

   2. Acetic acid = vinegar are used to highlight lesions

   3. Categorize lesions as
      a. Consistent with pap smear abnormality - yes or no
      b. Satisfactory visualization of lesion - yes or no
      c. Biopsy lesion and compare histology to pap smear

B. Endocervical curettage to evaluate cervix above colposcopic visualization

C. Cone biopsy - cold knife or loop excision or laser excision - specimen evaluated by pathologist
   1. Excision of entire transformation zone
   2. Required when unsatisfactory colposcopic exam
   3. Required when endocervical curettage has dysplastic cells present
   4. Required when colposcopic appearance worrisome for invasive cancer

D. Ablative therapy - no tissue sent to pathology - the procedure destroys transformation zone
   1. Cryotherapy - most common - least expensive
   2. Laser vaporization
   3. Requires satisfactory colposcopy - biopsy explains pap smear - endocervical curettage negative - no suspicion of cancer

IV. Clinical Presentation of Cervix Cancer

    A.   Premalignant disease - dysplasia
        1.   Asymptomatic
        2.   Cervix appears normal to naked eye
        3.   Can be detected by colposcopy
        4.   Can be detected by Lugol's staining

    B.   Invasive cancer symptoms
        1.   Postcoital bleeding - most specific symptom
        2.   Abnormal menstrual periods - intermenstrual bleeding or heavier periods
        3.   Postmenopausal bleeding
        4.   Abnormal discharge
        5.   Pain is a very late finding and usually signifies advanced disease

    C.   Biopsy of cervix required for diagnosis

    D.   Cone biopsy needed if entertaining diagnosis of Stage Ia

    E.   Pelvic exam, physical exam, chest x-ray and intravenous pyelogram needed for staging

V. Invasive Cervix Cancer - Staging - FIGO System - International Federation of Gynecology and Obstetrics

    A.   Rules of staging
        1.   Clinical exam is the basis of the stage - this is not a pathologic staging system

        2.   Radiologic procedures required
            a.   Intravenous pyelogram
            b.   Chest radiograph

        3.   Exams allowed
            a.   Cystoscopy
            b.   Proctoscopy

    B.   Stage I - tumor confirmed to cervix
        1.   Stage IA - tumor seen on cone biopsy or hysterectomy specimen to be no more than 5 mm deep and 7 mm wide

        2.   Stage IB - tumor larger than Stage IA but confined to the cervix

        3.   Stage IIA - tumor invades vagina but not lower 1/3

        4.   Stage IIB - tumor invades parametria but has not reached pelvic sidewall or created hydronephrosis

        5.   Stage IIIA - tumor extends to lower 1/3 of vagina

        6.   Stage IIIB - tumor has extended to pelvic sidewall or there is hydronephrosis

        7.   Stage IVA - spread of tumor to bladder or rectum confirmed by biopsy

        8.   Stage IVB - metastatic spread to distant site (i.e. supraclavicular node or lung metastasis)

VI. Treatment of Cervix Cancer

A. Stage IA
1. A subset of Stage IA patients with excellent prognostic features (i.e. less than 3 mm of invasion, no lymphatic or vascular invasion confluent tongues of tumor on cone biopsy) can be treated with a vaginal hysterectomy

2. Bad prognosis - patients should have radical hysterectomy and pelvic lymphadenectomy

B. Stage IB
1. Radical hysterectomy and pelvic lymphadenectomy is a treatment option
   a. Defined by the removal of uterus with its supporting ligaments the uterosacral and cardinal ligaments - to obtain good surgical margins around the tumor
   b. Requires dissection of lower 1/3 of ureter down to bladder
   c. Removal of all lymph nodes draining cervix = hypogastric obturator, external iliac and common iliac - para-aortic may also be removed
   d. Complications of radical hysterectomy
      1.) 1-2% urinary fistula
      2.) 20-30% bladder dysfunction including urinary retention

2. Radiation therapy can be used for Stage IB patients also and is the best choice for all higher stages

C. Radiation therapy
1. External beam radiation therapy or teletherapy is given as 180 rads or cGy daily Monday through Friday for 5 1/2 weeks until 5040 cGy is reached.

2. Brachytherapy - or intracavitary therapy - tandem in the cervix and ovoid in the vaginal fornices is generally given twice with 2000 cGy given each application.

3. Complications - less than 5% major complications
   a. Short-term
      1.) nausea
      2.) diarrhea
   b. Long-term
      1.) Radiation cystitis
      2.) Radiation proctitis
      3.) Vaginal vault necrosis
      4.) Fistula

VII. Five-year Survival of Cervix Cancer Patients

Stage IA	100%
Stage IB	85%
Stage IIA	70%
Stage IIB	65%
Stage III	30%

Five year survival for all stages combined is 50%

ENDOMETRIAL NEOPLASIA

I.   **Epidemiology and Risk Factors**

    A.   Fourth most common cancer in females

        1.   Approximately 33,000 new cases annually

        2.   Primarily a disease of postmenopausal females (75%)

            a.   Average age of onset is 60 years.

            b.   5% of cases occur in females younger than 40 years of age

        3.   In 75% of all cases, the tumor is confined to the uterine corpus.

    B.   Estrogen exposure

        1.   Endogenous

            a.   Obesity   > 30 lbs.   3 x increased risk

                                    > 50 lbs.   10 x increased risk

            b.   Late menopause (2.4x)/nulliparity (2x)

            c.   Anovulation

            d.   Estrogen secreting tumors

        2.   Exogenous - Unopposed estrogen replacement treatment

    C.   Hyperplasia

        1.   Simple - progression of cancer in 1% of cases

        2.   Complex - atypical - progression to cancer in 29% of cases

II.   **Prevention**

    A.   Treatment for complex atypical hyperplasia

        1.   Hysterectomy - treatment of choice in patients who have completed child bearing

        2.   High dose progestin therapy with periodic endometrial sampling in selected patients

    B.   Progestin therapy included with estrogen for hormonal replacement therapy

        1.   Progestin administered at least 10-14 days per month.

    C.   "Progesterone challenge test" (Gambrel)

        1.   Amenorrheic/hypermenorrheic perimenopausal patients

        2.   Any patient exposed to prolonged unopposed endogenous estrogen stimulation

III.   **Diagnosis**

    A.   Symptoms

        1.   90% of patients have abnormal vaginal discharge including 80% with abnormal bleeding.

2. Endometrial cells on cervical cytology in a postmenopausal woman should prompt the clinician to perform an endometrial biopsy.

B. Histologic assessment
1. Fractional dilatation & curettage

2. Endometrial biopsy - office procedure

3. Hysteroscopy and directed biopsy

C. Transvaginal ultrasound
1. Fewer than 10% of women with postmenopausal bleeding will have endometrial cancer.

2. Endometrial thickness < 5 mm can potentially spare sampling in 80% of women.

3. Recurrent bleeding after negative evaluation is an indication for hysteroscopy and/or curettage.

IV. Pathology

A. Endometrioid adenocarcinoma occurs in 75-80% of cases.

B. Grading varies from well-differentiated (Grade I) to poorly differentiated (Grade III).
1. Advanced grade is associated with higher risk of deep myometrial invasion and lymph node involvement (para-aortic and pelvic)

C. Papillary serous and clear cell histologic types are associated with aggressive biologic behavior.

V. Staging

A. Staging is performed surgically and includes TAH/BSO, pelvic/para-aortic lymph node sampling (with specific indications) and peritoneal cytology.

B.   Corpus Cancer Surgical Staging, FIGO 1988

Stages	Characteristics
IA G123	Tumor limited to endometrium
IB G123	Invasion to <1/2 myometrium
IC G123	Invasion to >1/2 myometrium
IIA G123	Endocervical glandular involvement only
IIB G123	Cervical stromal invasion
IIIA G123	Tumor invades serosa or adnexae or positive peritoneal cytology
IIIB G123	Vaginal metastases
IIIC G123	Metastases to pelvic or para-aortic lymph nodes
IVA G123	Tumor invasion bladder and/or bowel mucosa
IVB	Distant metastases including intra-abdominal and/or inguinal lymph node

HISTOPATHOLOGY - DEGREE OF DIFFERENTIATION

Cases should be grouped by the degree of differentiation of the adenocarcinoma:
- G1   5% or less of a nonsquamous or nonmorular solid growth pattern
- G2   6%-50% of a nonsquamous or nonmorular solid growth pattern
- G3   More than 50% of a nonsquamous or nonmorular solid growth pattern

NOTES ON PATHOLOGIC GRADING

Notable nuclear atypia, inappropriate for the architectural grade, raises the grade of a grade I or grade II tumor by 1.

In serous adenocarcinomas, clear cell adenocarcinomas, and squamous cell carcinomas, nuclear grading takes precedence.

Adenocarcinomas with squamous differentiation are graded according to the nuclear grade of the glandular component.

RULES RELATED TO STAGING

Because corpus cancer is now surgically staged, procedures previously used for determination of stages are no longer applicable, such as the finding of fractional D&C to differentiate between stage I and II.

It is appreciated that there may be a small number of patients with corpus cancer who will be treated primarily with radiation therapy. If that is the case, the clinical staging adopted by FIGO in 1971 would still apply but designation of that staging system would be noted.

Ideally, width of the myometrium should be measured along with the width of tumor invasion.

OVARIAN NEOPLASIA

I.   Differential Diagnosis of Pelvic Masses

    A.   Gynecologic
        1.   Ovary-Neoplasm (benign or malignant), functional cyst, endometriosis

        2.   Fallopian tube - tubo-ovarian abscess, ectopic pregnancy, hydrosalpinx, malignancy

        3.   Uterus - pregnancy, fibroids (especially pedunculated)

    B.   Non-gynecologic
        1.   Bowel - feces, diverticulitis, appendicitis, colon cancer

        2.   Urinary - distended bladder, pelvic kidney, urachal cyst

        3.   Miscellaneous - retroperitoneal neoplasm, abdominal wall mass

II.   Evaluation of Pelvic Mass

    A.   Ultrasound - transabdominal or transvaginal ultrasound to help identify origin of mass. Solid or solid cystic ovarian masses, with internal papillations, thick septa, and ascites are characteristic of malignancy

    B.   Serum B-hCG - for menstruate women to rule out ectopic or intrauterine pregnancy

    C.   Serum CA-125 - If elevated, highly predictive of malignancy in post menopausal women. Limited value in premenopausal women due to false positives (endometriosis, pregnancy, infection, menses, leiomyoma, etc.). Normal CA125 does not exclude malignancy.

    D.   Barium enema - helpful in ruling out bowel malignancy

    E.   IVP - rule out pelvic kidney, establish course of ureters

III.   Management of Ovarian Mass

    A.   Reproductive age women
        1.   Cystic mass, $\leq$ 8 cm - expectant management with re-examination in 6 - 8 weeks (after menstrual cycle). May consider suppression with oral contraceptives. 70% will resolve indicating functional cyst. 30% will have persistent or enlarged mass requiring operative intervention.

        2.   Mass > 8 cm or solid/cystic - requires operative intervention

    B.   Premenarchal or postmenopausal - ovarian masses generally require operative evaluation

IV. Ovarian Cancer

A. Epidemiology
   1. 1-2% of women develop ovarian cancer

   2. Sharp rise at age 40 (peak incidence age 50-55)

   3. Approximately 20,000 new cases and 12,000 deaths from ovarian cancer in U.S. every year (fifth leading cause of cancer death in women- leading gynecologic cause of death)

B. Risk factors
   1. Increased risk - industrialization, dietary, increased ovulation, familial (approximately 1-5% of ovarian cancers may be genetically determined)

   2. Decreased risk - oral contraceptives, pregnancy, lactation

C. Screening
   1. American Cancer Society guidelines annual pelvic exam after age 40
   2. Ultrasound and tumor markers - not proven cost effective

D. Histology

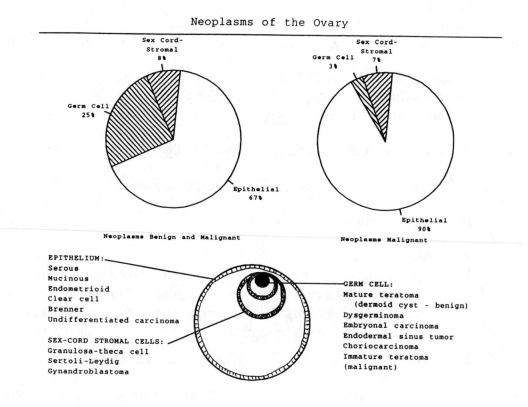

Neoplasms of the Ovary

Sex Cord-Stromal 8%
Germ Cell 25%
Epithelial 67%
Neoplasms Benign and Malignant

Sex Cord-Stromal 7%
Germ Cell 3%
Epithelial 90%
Neoplasms Malignant

EPITHELIUM:
Serous
Mucinous
Endometrioid
Clear cell
Brenner
Undifferentiated carcinoma

SEX-CORD STROMAL CELLS:
Granulosa-theca cell
Sertoli-Leydig
Gynandroblastoma

GERM CELL:
Mature teratoma
 (dermoid cyst - benign)
Dysgerminoma
Embryonal carcinoma
Endodermal sinus tumor
Choriocarcinoma
Immature teratoma
(malignant)

E. FIGO Stage for Primary Carcinoma of the Ovary (1987)

Stage I   Growth limited to the ovaries.

Stage IA   Growth limited to one ovary; no ascites. No tumor on the external surface; capsule intact.

Stage IB   Growth limited to both ovaries; no ascites. No tumor on the external surface; capsule intact.

Stage IC   Tumor either Stage IA or IB but with tumor on the surface of one or both ovaries; or with capsule ruptured; or with ascites present containing malignant cells or with positive peritoneal washings.

Stage II   Growth involving one or both ovaries with pelvic extension.

Stage IIA   Extension and/or metastasis to the uterus and/or tubes.

Stage IIB   Extension to other pelvic tissues.

Stage IIC*   Tumor either Stage IIA or IIB but with tumor on the surface of one or both ovaries; or with capsule ruptured; or with ascites present containing malignant cells or with positive peritoneal washings.

Stage III   Tumor involving one or both ovaries with peritoneal implants outside the pelvis and/or positive retroperitoneal or inguinal nodes. Superficial liver metastasis equals Stage III. Tumor is limited to the true pelvis but with histologically verified malignant extension to small bowel or omentum.

Stage IIIA   Tumor grossly limited to the true pelvis with negative nodes but with histologically confirmed microscopic seeding of abdominal peritoneal surfaces.

Stage IIIB   Tumor of one or both ovaries with histologically confirmed implants of abdominal peritoneal surfaces, none exceeding 2 cm in diameter. Nodes negative.

Stage IIIC   Abdominal implants greater than 2 cm in diameter and/or positive retroperitoneal or inguinal nodes.

Stage IV   Growth involving one or both ovaries with distant metastasis. If pleural effusion is present there must be positive cytologic test results to allot a case to Stage IV. Parenchymal liver metastasis equals Stage IV.

* In order to evaluate the impact on prognosis of the different criteria for allotting cases to Stage IC or IIC, it would be of value to know if rupture of the capsule was spontaneous or caused by the surgeon, and if the source of the malignant cells detected was from peritoneal washings or ascites.

F. Management
    1. Surgery - staging and cytoreductive surgery
    2. Adjuvant therapy - stage IA, grade 1 tumors do not require adjuvant therapy, more advanced and higher grade lesions require further treatment.
        a. Chemotherapy - most commonly used (Cisplatin, Carboplatin, Cytoxan, Taxol)
        b. Radiotherapy - intraperitoneal P32 for early stage disease. Whole abdominal radiotherapy can be considered for more advanced diseases.

GESTATIONAL TROPHOBLASTIC DISEASE

I. **Presentation** - Diagnosis made with pelvic ultrasound, BhCG titers and computerized tomography (CT) scan may be necessary

   A. Hydatidiform mole presents with vaginal bleeding, passage of tissue or abnormal uterine growth during prenatal exams

   B. Invasive moles are diagnosed when evacuation of hydatidiform mole does not cause resolution of the beta human chorionic gonadotropin (βHCG)

   C. Placental site trophoblastic tumor usually presents with abnormal bleeding after term delivery and a persistent low βHCG level

   D. Choriocarcinoma - symptoms depend on metastatic sites
      1. Brain - seizures, coma
      2. Lung - hemoptysis
      3. Liver - right upper quadrant pain
      4. Vagina - mass or bleeding
      5. Uterus - vaginal bleeding

II. **Hydatidiform Mole** - Classic Ultrasound Characteristic is a Snowstorm Pattern

   A. Complete mole
      1. Abnormal pregnancy composed entirely of hydropic (fluid-filled, edematous) villi, with hyperplastic trophoblasts

      2. No fetal parts or fetal red blood cells seen

      3. Capable of invasion and malignant transformation into choriocarcinoma

      4. Secretes βHCG

      5. 20% require chemotherapy for cure

   B. Partial mole
      1. Hydropic villi present
      2. Fetal component present
      3. Fetal RBCs
      4. Less likely to need chemotherapy

   C. Treatment
      1. Suction dilation and curettage (D&C)

      2. No therapy needed for theca lutein cysts in ovaries - they resolve spontaneously

      3. Be prepared for pulmonary complications secondary to deportation of villi to lungs

      4. Hyperthyroidism and preeclampsia are possible complications

   D.   Follow-up
        1.   Weekly human chorionic gonadotropin (βHCG) until normal

        2.   Then monthly for three months

        3.   Then every other month

        4.   Oral contraception for one year

        5.   Pregnancy allowed after one year without recurrence

III.   Invasive Mole

   A.   Diagnosis made by HCG plateau or rise after evacuation of hydatidiform mole

   B.   Histologic diagnosis not necessary

   C.   Ultrasound of uterus to be sure it is not new pregnancy

   D.   Chemotherapy - single agent Methotrexate or Actinomycin D

   E.   Hysterectomy is treatment alternative for noncompliant patient or older women who has completed childbearing

IV.   Classification of Gestational Trophoblastic Neoplasia

   A.   Non metastatic - confined to uterus

   B.   Metastatic - good prognosis
        1.   Usually lung metastasis
        2.   Less than four months since the antecedent pregnancy
        3.   HCG < 40,000
        4.   No metastasis to brain or liver
        5.   No prior chemotherapy

   C.   Metastatic - poor prognosis
        1.   Antecedent term pregnancy
        2.   Brain or liver metastasis
        3.   High HCG > 40,000
        4.   Previous chemotherapy
        5.   Requires aggressive multi-agent chemotherapy
        6.   Usually give radiation to brain or liver

ETHICS AND LEGAL ISSUES

ETHICS IN OBSTETRICS AND GYNECOLOGY

I. Introduction

A. Ethics in the broad perspective concerns distinguishing right from wrong and acting accordingly. In medicine, ethics concerns the physician making decisions that are best for the patient. In obstetrics, where there is concern for two patients, ethical decisions may be more complex and difficult.

II. Beneficence

A. Concern for the patient's interest is called beneficence, and requires that the physician:
1. evaluate the patient's clinical problem
2. outline the various options for treatment to improve the problem
3. choose the treatment plan that offers the greatest chance of success with the least amount of risk.

III. Autonomy: Informed Consent

A. Autonomy is the concept that the patient has the right to make her own decisions. Once the clinical problem has been evaluated and the decision made as to the best plan of management, the physician is obligated to explain the situation and to review each treatment on with the patient, explaining the benefits and risks of each. The process is called informed consent. The patient's permission is required before embarking on any treatment. The patient has the right to accept or not accept the physician's recommendations.

B Beneficence and autonomy are always present in the doctor-patient relationship. In most medical situations their presence is assumed: if the doctor prescribes a medicine or treatment, the mere fact that the patient takes the medicine or undergoes the treatment implies that the patient accepted the physicians beneficence and yielded none of his or her autonomy by undergoing the treatment. It is only when there is conflict in their relationship that ethical concepts are called into play.

C. An example of conflict is the case of a young married woman, mother of 3 small children, who is found to have a stage III squamous carcinoma of the cervix. The physician recommends diation therapy. The patient refuses because she is afraid of being "burned". Usually such a conflict can be resolved by further discussion with other physicians, members of the patient's family, other patients who have had radiation therapy, etc...

IV. The Abortion Conflict

A. Dr. Daniel Callahan has referred to the abortion conflict as a "chronic public illness." He continues on to point out that the conflict has gone beyond a debate to become so polarized that there simply is no middle ground, no room at all for compromise.

B. However the conflict is settled (if it ever is), each physician must develop his or her own method of dealing with the issue of abortion as it relates to the physician's own set of moral beliefs and the practice of medicine and to the needs of the patient. It is not enough for the individual physician to have decided whether he or she is "pro-choice" or "pro-life", or whether he or she will perform abortions themselves. It is also necessary for each physician to face the issue of how to advise his or her patients when their needs are in conflict with the moral and ethical beliefs of the physician. The major conflict arises when the stated needs of the patient includes a legal abortion and the physician is "pro-life". To apply the principle of beneficence to the doctor-patient relationship, the "pro-life physician" finds himself or herself in a difficult ethical situation. Such a conflict can only be dealt with appropriately in a non-confrontational, non emotional setting with the doctor-patient ship continuing to be based on the beneficence of the physician and the autonomy of the patient. As in other clinical relationships, the physician is to evaluate the clinical situation and make recommendations to the patient, respecting the patient's right to accept or refuse the recommendation. Physicians must allow the patient to know the physician's personal beliefs particularly if those beliefs interfere with a full discussion of treatment options with the patient. Each physician should intellectually consider this situation and how he or she is going to react to it <u>before it arises in a true clinical situation</u>.

V. The Fetus as a Patient

A. Until recently the fetus was considered only a potential heir or person; as such the fetus was not a citizen and had no "rights" as a citizen until it was born alive. While in most legal jurisdictions the fetus is not a <u>person</u> or a <u>citizen</u>, recent medical practice treats the fetus as a <u>patient</u>, whose best interests are to be considered when making obstetrical decisions. Indeed, concern for fetal welfare routinely results in the physician recommending and the mother accepting the increased risk of cesarean section even when it is performed solely for fetal indications.

B   .Recent advances in medical science and imaging have enabled the physician to diagnose and directly treat individual fetuses. With the possible exception of fetal intraperitoneal or intravascular transfusions or administration of steroids to the mother to stimulate development of fetal lung maturity, invasive fetal therapy remains experimental. As such, experimental therapy need not be discussed as an option unless the patient continues to insist upon exhausting all possibilities.

VI. Access to Care:

A   .The ideal of American Medicine is that care should be available to all regardless of race, creed, place of residence or ability to pay. It is clear that some citizens have more access to care than others. Except in very remote areas, most American citizens have access to medical care at some level. Access is one thing, but paying for it is another. It is clear that the physician or hospital that receives less reimbursement for services than it costs to give them, will soon lose the ability to provide medical care at all. Most developed countries consider medical care a "right" of its citizens, ,and many have systems that feature universal access and coverage for medical care. In every system, however, there are restrictions on expenditures so that the system can remain financially sound enough to continue to provide at least minimum services to all. Recent increases in the age of the population, expensive technological advances and demand for services threaten nearly every national economy in the developed world.

B. Ethical considerations arise when there is conflict between a need for medical care and the inability of the patient to pay for it. The ideal of beneficence is strained when we must decide between a very expensive transplant procedure for an individual or the provision of less costly preventive care for a large number of individuals. For instance prenatal care for hundreds of women can be obtained for the cost of a single liver transplant, with the probability of "saving" more than one life. The more demand there is for decreasing funds for government expenditures for medical care, the more debate there will be concerning the relationship between cost and benefit for individuals as well as society in general.

C. Cost/benefit relationships in medicine usually follow a hyperbolic curve. It is clear that those technologies offering the greatest benefit at the lowest cost (the left side of the curve) should be pursued more than those that have high cost and little added benefit (on the right side of the curve). Preventive medicine, i.e., immunizations or improved sanitation, tend to fall to the left, while high technology diagnostic and therapeutic procedures tend to fall on the right side of the curve

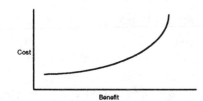

D. The physician faced with an ethical conflict in patient care would do well to follow the medical golden rule: "Do unto your patients as you would want done to you under the same circumstances".

VII. Assisted Reproductive Technology

A. Extension of the technological advance of in vitro fertilization using the wife's ova and her husband's sperm to the use of frozen ova, blastocysts and non-related people's gametes and he use of surrogate uteri have created widely discussed dilemmas. The majority of these dilemmas are legal rather than strictly ethical. It would seem that both beneficence and autonomy are properly served when each of the participants are properly informed and give their consent. Strictly ethical considerations arise when more zygotes or fetuses than desired are produced in the effort to make each fertilization attempt likely to be as successful as possible. Donation of unwanted "left over" frozen ova or zygotes to another person (properly informed as to potential consequences) would be beneficent for the parents, as well as the donors. Outright destruction of such unwanted human material might not be beneficent, but it is apparently legal in most jurisdictions.

LEGAL ISSUES IN OBSTETRICS AND GYNECOLOGY

All physicians have certain rights and obligations concerning patient care.

I. Physician's Rights

A. Contracts

As with any private individual, physicians have the freedom not to enter into contracts if they do not wish to do so. Thus, physicians need not accept a given patient for care, and in theory, at least, do not have to even give a reason for the decision. In practice, however, physicians often have a legal requirement to care for whomever requests care: For instance, physicians often agree to accept the responsibility to be on call for various services. As a consequence of your hospital or practice affiliation agreements written or orally agreed to, i.e., emergency room or taking call for another the handicapped place physicians under obligations many of them do not realize they have. Generally speaking these laws prevent physicians from refusing care to patients with any type of handicap including highly infectious disease (such as AIDS), whether or not the patient has any opportunity to pay for care.

II. Patient's Rights (Physicians Obligations)

A. The Doctor-Patient Relationship

Although a written contract is rarely executed, a contract is implied when a patient seeks the services of a physician and the physician accepts the patient for care. The implied contract usually begins when the patient and the physician meet in a medical setting. In some cases, merely having the patient's name registered for an appointment has satisfied the requirement for a valid contract. Once the relationship is established, the doctor has the duty to provide such care as the ordinarily competent physician would provide under similar circumstances. The physician also has the duty to suggest a referral or consultation when he/she knows or ought to know, that he/she does not possess the requisite skill or knowledge for proper treatment. It should be pointed out, however, that the physician may limit the therapeutic relationship to include only certain areas of his/her expertise, and to limit his/her availability to certain times or places. However, unless clearly stated and understood by the patient, the physician had the duty to either be available for care of the patient should the need arise, or provide some other physician of equal skill and training to accept the responsibility for his patients when he/she is unavailable.

B. Informed Consent

Each patient has the right to be clearly informed as to all of the risks and all of the benefits of any treatment the physician proposes, including the risks and benefits of not having the suggested treatment or no treatment at all.

Each adult person has autonomy -- the right to make decisions for themselves— as long as those decisions do not harm other persons. When deciding upon a surgical or medical therapy, every patient has the right to refuse such therapy, or to chose an alternative regardless of the physicians recommendations.

Pregnancy: When the patient is pregnant, it is generally accepted that the mother will protect the interests of her fetus, and thus is expected to be able to make decisions about therapy that affect both her and the fetus, i.e., cesarean section. Since the Roe v. Wade decision allowing all women the right to abortion during the first trimester of pregnancy, however, some have concluded that the mother may not always act in the best interest of her fetus. Thus, where the decision of the mother seems to conflict with what seems to be the best interests of the fetus, conflict over therapy may arise. These are rare circumstances, and usually arise in an acute situation, i.e., refusal of emergency cesarean section for apparent fetal distress. As such, it may be impossible to find a solution to the conflict. It is clear, however, that in most states, the fetus is not a citizen and the mother is. Operating upon her against her will constitutes "battery" (negligent use of force by one person against another). Battery is a serious crime - a felony which may be punishable by imprisonment.

C. Confidentiality. Physicians must maintain confidentiality of whatever their patients tell them and whatever diseases or problems the physician discovers or suspects the patient to have. Thus, physicians are prohibited from revealing anything about their patients in public without specific permission to do so from the patient. In most instances, such permission is assumed when a treating physician discusses the patient's care with another physician who also is caring or going to care for or consult on the patient's care with the physician. A general rule to follow is that sharing of the patient's personal and medical information may be discussed with another person -- usually another physician -- when that sharing of information will be held in confidence by the other person and it will be in the best interests of the patient for the information to be shared.

D. Abandonment

Abandonment is the unilateral severance of the relationship between the physician and the patient, when continued medical attention is still necessary. It is clear that the patient who finds access to the physician denied may feel differently than the physician about whether medical attention continues to be needed. Thus, it is best for the physician who wants to terminate the physician-patient relationship do so in writing, giving the patient adequate time to find another physician (usually a few weeks is reasonable). Usually it is also helpful to supply a short list of other physicians the physician feels would be capable of providing any care needed.

E. Fraud

Medical care is based on trust. Physicians are trusted to act in their patient's best interests and to be honest in all dealings relating to medical practice. Fraud (a deception deliberately practiced to obtain unfair or unlawful gain) is decidedly unethical. The use of fraudulent claims for reimbursement from patients or insurance companies is unlawful. Deliberate misrepresentations of the efficacy of medical treatment is fraudulent. Since the public usually holds professional practitioners to a higher standard of behavior, physicians must be careful to avoid the slightest hint of fraud, deceit or lack of honesty.

MEDICAL MALPRACTICE

Medical malpractice is defined as negligent care that causes an injury. The plaintiff (the injured patient) must show that:

1.   There was a doctor-patient relationship between he/she and the accused physician (the defendant).

2.   The physician's care fell below the "standard of care", which is defined as that level of care that a prudent physician would have given in the same or similar circumstances.

3.   The plaintiff must prove that an injury occurred to him or her, and that

4.   The injury was caused by the negligence of the physician.

Since an increasing number of claims have been filed in recent years most physicians obtain malpractice insurance. Malpractice insurance insures the physician against the costs of his/her defense (lawyers fees, expert witness fees, court costs, etc...) as well as money awarded to the plaintiff by the court or the settlement of the case out of court. The amount of insurance coverage is limited and varies with the cost of the insurance, the malpractice "climate" of the region where the physician practices and the type of policy.

There are two general types of medical malpractice insurance:

a.   "Occurrence". With occurrence policies the physician is covered for any malpractice claim that arose from an injury that occurred during any time that the physician was insured, whether or not the physician now has insurance with the same or any other company.

b.   "Claims made". This type of insurance covers the physician only if the policy is in force when the event occurs and when the claim is made.

The premiums for "claims made" policies are generally initially less than "occurrence" policies, but when the physician wishes to retire or move, he/she must continue to pay an annual premium or purchase a special larger broader policy to cover all claims made until the physician's death. This payment is referred to as "the tail". The expense of purchasing "the tail" is ordinarily large enough to inhibit the physician's plans to move out of the region covered by his insurance company or to retire.

The Malpractice Suit

To receive a "summons" from the court that accuses you of malpractice is devastating for most physicians. The following is a general overview of a typical case:

1.   The patient seeks an attorney and makes a complaint.

2.   The attorney evaluates merits of the case by reviewing the medical records. Before officially filing a malpractice claim, the attorney must become convinced that the patient's claim meets the criteria for malpractice.

3.   A claim is filed with the court.

4. The court notifies the physician that a claim has been filed.

5. The insured physician should notify his/her malpractice insurance company.

6. The malpractice insurance company will require a summary of the case from the physician and a copy of all pertinent records. Many physicians choose to involve their personal attorney as well as that chosen by the malpractice carrier.

7. Depositions. Once the basic information is available, the plaintiff's attorney will want to interview you about what you did, why you did it, how did the injury occur, etc... This interview is called a deposition. It is done under oath, and a court reporter transcribes the proceedings. Your attorneys (the insurance carrier and your personal attorney) will be there. You will meet with them before the deposition to go over the facts and strategy. Other witnesses (nurses, doctors) may also be deposed by the plaintiff's attorney.

    You and these witnesses are "fact" witnesses, and are responsible only to testify as to what you saw and did and why you acted in the way you did. Fact witnesses are required to respond when subpoenaed, as a subpoena is an order of the court. If you fail to respond you may be held in contempt of court and subjected to fines or other punishment.

8. Expert witnesses. Experts are "opinion" witnesses called to establish standards of care or cause of the injury. The plaintiff's expert often will differ in his opinions from the experts your attorneys consult.

9. Trial. After all the information is gathered and the plaintiff's attorney understands as much as possible about the merit of the plaintiff's case, the case is brought to trial. (Unless the case can be "settled" to the satisfaction of both parties.) Many malpractice cases are dropped by the plaintiff or settled prior to trial. During the trial the plaintiff will tell his/her story, and other witnesses may be brought in to substantiate it. Your attorneys have the right to "cross examine" each witness to question various points. After the plaintiff has presented his/her side, your attorneys will question you and your expert witnesses under oath, answering all claims made against you.

The trial situation is complicated. Your responsibilities are to tell the truth at all times, and be responsive to the advice of your attorneys.

Doctor's "win" most malpractice cases.

REVIEW QUESTIONS & ANSWERS

QUESTIONS

1. The false negative rate for PAP smears is
    a.   < 1 %
    b.   5 - 10 %
    c.   15 - 40 %
    d.   50 - 60 %
    e.   70 - 80 %

2. Risk factors for cervical dysplasia include all of the following EXCEPT
    a.   multiple sexual partners
    b.   early age of first intercourse
    c.   circumcised partner
    d.   cigarette smoking
    e.   in-utero DES exposure

3. A twenty year old is found to have moderate dysplasia (high grade SIL) on a routine PAP. Moderate inflammation is noted on the PAP. The next appropriate step in management is
    a.   Repeat PAP in 3 months
    b.   Treat inflammation and repeat PAP in 3 months
    c.   Colposcopy and biopsies
    d.   Wire loop excision of the transformation zone
    e.   Cold knife conization

4. Advantages of laser ablation of the cervix over cryotherapy for dysplasia include
    a.   better success rate
    b.   lower risk of bleeding
    c.   lower cost
    d.   all of the above
    e.   none of the above

Match the following descriptions with their definitions
    5.   Urethrocele
    6.   Cystocele
    7.   Rectocele
    8.   Enterocoele
    9.   Procidentia

    a.   Bulge in the lower third of the vagina overlying the urethra
    b.   Bulge in anterior wall of vagina
    c.   Herniation through the pouch of Douglas
    d.   Prolapse of cervix and uterus
    e.   Bulge in posterior vaginal wall

Match the following
    a.   Post partum blues
    b.   Post partum depression
    c.   Post partum psychosis

    10.   Occurrence rate < 0.3 %
    11.   Initial treatment with tricyclic antidepressants
    12.   Usually occurs 48 - 72 hours post partum
    13.   Manifested by feelings of alienation from the baby

Match the following with their average age
    14.   Menarche
    15.   Growth spurt
    16.   Thelarche
    17.   Adrenarche

    a.   9.5
    b.   10.5
    c.   11
    d.   11.5
    e.   12.8

Match the following types of precocious puberty with their definitions
    18.   Isosexual
    19.   True
    20.   Pseudo
    21.   Heterosexual

    a.   Premature activation of hypothalamic - pituitary - gonadal axis by GnRH pulses
    b.   Inappropriate for genetic sex
    c.   Appropriate for genetic sex
    d.   Not dependent on GnRH pulses

22.   Etiologies of precocious puberty include all of the following EXCEPT
    a.   CNS tumor
    b.   McCune Albright syndrome
    c.   Hypothyroidism
    d.   Adrenal hyperplasia
    e.   Klinefelter's syndrome

23.   The predominate flora in the normal vagina is
    a.   Lactobacilli
    b.   Bacteroides
    c.   Peptostreptococcus
    d.   Gardnerella vaginalis

24.　The normal vaginal pH is
　　a.　3.5 - 3.9
　　b.　4.0 - 4.4
　　c.　4.5 - 5.0
　　d.　5.1 - 5.5
　　e.　5.6 - 7.0

25.　The etiology of primary dysmenorrhea is most commonly
　　a.　excess prostaglandin production
　　b.　development of uterine myomas
　　c.　endometriosis
　　d.　adenomyosis
　　e.　endometrial polyps

26.　The most effective over the counter treatment for dysmenorrhea is
　　a.　Acetaminophen
　　b.　Aspirin
　　c.　Ibuprofen
　　d.　Acetaminophen/caffeine combination
　　e.　Aspirin/caffeine combination

27.　Adenomyosis can be diagnosed by
　　a.　Physical examination
　　b.　Endometrial biopsy
　　c.　Transvaginal Ultrasound
　　d.　Hysterosalpingogram
　　e.　Histologic examination of uterus

28.　Endometriosis can be diagnosed by
　　a.　symptoms
　　b.　pelvic ultrasound
　　c.　serum CA - 125
　　d.　serum anti endometrial antibodies
　　e.　direct visualization of lesions

Match the following adult structures with their embryonal precursor

29. Ovary
30. Round Ligament
31. Lower vagina
32. Clitoris
33. Fallopian tube
34. Clitoris
35. Labia minora
36. Gartners duct cyst

a. Gubernaculum
b. Mesonephric (Wolffian) duct
c. Paramesonephric (Mullerian) duct
d. Genital ridge
e. Urogenital folds
f. Genital tubercle
g. Urogenital sinus

Match the following presentations of a pelvic mass with the appropriate management

37. 6 cm cystic mass in a 29 year old
38. 9 cm cystic mass in a 29 year old
39. 6 cm cystic/solid mass in a 29 year old
40. 6 cm cystic mass in a 6 year old
41. 6 cm cystic mass in a 69 year old

a. Observation and reexamination in 6 -8 weeks
b. Operative intervention
c. Draw CA 125 and base management decision on results
d. Draw CA 125 and operative intervention

42. At laparotomy, a woman is found to have ovarian cancer involving both ovaries. There are multiple 1 to 2 cm implants over the pelvic peritoneum, and the periaortic and pelvic nodes are negative. The stage would be
   A. II B
   B. III A
   C. III B
   D. III C
   E. IV

43. Characteristics of a partial molar pregnancy include
   A. Absence of nucleated RBC
   B. Absence of hydropic villi
   C. Absence of fetal component
   D. Increased malignant potential
   E. None of the above

44. Characteristics of poor prognosis metastatic gestational trophoblastic disease include all of the following EXCEPT
   A. Antecedent term pregnancy
   B. Lung metastasis
   C. HCG > 40,000
   D. Previous chemotherapy
   E. Brain or liver metastasis

45. Which of the following is least likely to be associated with vulvar carcinoma at presentation?
   A. Vulvar condyloma
   B. Lichen sclerosis
   C. Hyperplastic vulvar dystrophy
   D. Mixed dystrophy
   E. Vulvar intraepithelial neoplasia

46. A biopsy of a 2 cm lesion of the vulva shows squamous cell carcinoma. There is a fixed hard node in the ipsilateral inguinal chain and no evidence of distant metastasis. The stage would be
   A. I (T1N0M0)
   B. II (T2N0M0)
   C. III (T3N0M0)
   D. III (T1N1M0)
   E. III (T2N1M0)

47. Endometrial carcinoma with invasion of > 1/2 of the myometrium, negative node biopsies and no invasion of the cervix would be stage
   A. I A
   B. I B
   C. I C
   D. II A
   E. II B

48. All of the following are risk factors for endometrial carcinoma EXCEPT
   A. Obesity
   B. Nulliparity
   C. Late menopause
   D. Combination estrogen/progestin hormone therapy
   E. Anovulation

49. Positive evidence of pregnancy is established by:
   A. Cessation of menses
   B. Congestion of the vagina
   C. Positive urine test for beta hCG
   D. Positive blood test for beta hCG
   E. Demonstration of the fetal heart

50. The most reliable clinical estimator of gestational age is:
   A. Date of the last menstrual period in a normally cycling woman
   B. Ultrasound determination at 32 weeks
   C. Date of first auscultation of the fetal heart
   D. Date of first perception of fetal movements
   E. Physical examination at 12 weeks of gestation

51. During normal pregnancy, the uterus first becomes palpable in the lower abdomen at:
   A. 8 weeks
   B. 12 weeks
   C. 16 weeks
   D. 20 weeks
   E. 24 weeks

52. Evaluations to be determined at each prenatal visit include all of the following EXCEPT:
   A. Weight
   B. Blood pressure
   C. Hemoglobin determination
   D. Ascertainment of fetal heart tones
   E. Urine dipstick for protein and glucose

53. Average weight gain in a normal pregnancy should be:
   A. 10 pounds
   B. 20 pounds
   C. 30 pounds
   D. 40 pounds
   E. 50 pounds

54. All of the following are true statements about advanced maternal age in pregnancy EXCEPT:
   A. 6% of births in the United States are among women age 35 or older
   B. Advanced maternal age appears to carry a greater risk of spontaneous abortion
   C. Advanced maternal age appears to carry an increased risk of chromosomal abnormalities
   D. Women of advanced maternal age are at lower risk for cesarean section
   E. Advanced maternal age is associated with a greater risk of hypertension

55. A 35-year old women presents with no menses for six months. Her serum prolactin is normal. She does not have withdrawal bleeding after progesterone. She does have bleeding after a combined estrogen and progestin treatment and her serum FSH is 100. The most likely diagnosis is:
   A. Outflow tract obstruction
   B. Asherman's Syndrome
   C. Hyperprolactinemia
   D. Premature menopause
   E. Hypogonadotrophic hypogonadism

56. A 28-year old woman presents with secondary amenorrhea of six months duration. After a history and physical and after pregnancy has been excluded, the next step should be:
    A. Measurement of a TSH and prolactin and administer progestational challenge
    B. Measurement of gonadotropin assay and progestational challenge
    C. Measurement of gonadotrophin assay followed by a 21-day cycle of estrogen and progestin
    D. Measurement of chromosomes and gonadotrophin level
    E. Measurement of gonadotrophins and a coronal CT scan

57. An 18-year old presents with primary amenorrhea. Physical exam reveals a lack of secondary sex characteristics and the presence of a uterus. Which of the following is NOT a possible diagnosis?
    A. Sawyer's Syndrome
    B. 17 hydroxylase deficiency
    C. Turner's Syndrome
    D. Rokitansky Custer Hauser Syndrome
    E. Pure XY gonadal dysgenesis

58. The pain pathway from the uterus and cervix is carried through:
    A. T4 through T6
    B. T7 through T9
    C. T10 through L1
    D. L2 through S1
    E. S2 through S4

59. The pain pathways from the vagina and perineum are carried through
    A. T4 through T6
    B. T7 through T9
    C. T10 through L1
    D. L2 through S1
    E. S2 through S4

60. The most common method of contraception in the United States is:
    A. Sterilization
    B. Oral contraceptives
    C. Intrauterine device
    D. Barrier methods
    E. Injectable contraceptives

61. Which of the following is the most effective method of contraception?
    A. Oral contraceptives
    B. Diaphragm
    C. Condoms
    D. Norplant
    E. Intrauterine device

62. Match the landmark sign with the earliest menstrual gestational age:

_____Positive radioimmunoassay of hCG   A.   4 weeks

_____Amplified fetal heart tones heard   B.   12 weeks

_____Fundal height (cm)   C.   16 weeks

_____Maternal perception of fetal movement   D.   20 weeks

    E.   24 weeks

63. Which vitamin or mineral supplement is routinely recommended during pregnancy?
    A.   Iron
    B.   Calcium
    C.   Fluoride
    D.   Folic acid
    E.   Vitamin B6

64. Advanced maternal age is associated with a greater risk of all of the following EXCEPT:
    A.   Stillbirth
    B.   Pre-eclampsia
    C.   Cesarean section
    D.   Placental abruption
    E.   Spontaneous abortion

65. Routine screening during pregnancy is not recommended for which type of infection?
    A.   Gonorrhea
    B.   Rubella
    C.   Chlamydia
    D.   Hepatitis B
    E.   Bacterial vaginosis

66. Uterine contractions adequate to cause cervical change would be expected to have the following characteristic:
    A.   Frequency every 4 minutes with duration of 45 seconds
    B.   Frequency every 2 minutes with duration of 30 seconds
    C.   Frequency every 3 minutes with duration of 45 seconds
    D.   Frequency every 3 minutes with duration of 60 seconds
    E.   Frequency every 5 minutes with duration of 75 seconds

67. A. nulliparous patient at 41 weeks has adequate contractions. For the past three hours, her cervix dilated from 5 cm to 6 cm and the presenting part descended 1 cm. The labor pattern would be described as being:
    A. Normal
    B. Protraction disorder
    C. An arrest of second stage
    D. A prolonged latent phase
    E. An arrest of active phase

68. The most appropriate treatment for the above case would be:
    A. Expectant therapy
    B. Oxytocin infusion
    C. A cesarean section
    D. A vacuum application
    E. Subcutaneous terbutaline

69. The proper order for mechanisms of normal labor is:
    A. Descent, flexion, extension, internal rotation
    B. Flexion, descent, internal rotation, extension
    C. Extension, internal rotation, flexion, descent
    D. Internal rotation, descent, extension, flexion
    E. Descent, extension, internal rotation, flexion

70. The proper order of events for the vaginal delivery of a cephalically-presenting fetus is:
    A. Upward traction of head, external head rotation, allow crowning, suction of upper airway, delivery of anterior shoulder
    B. Allow crowning, external head rotation, suction of upper airway, delivery of anterior shoulder, upward traction of head

71. The most common indication for a cesarean section is:
    A. Repeat cesarean
    B. Failure to progress
    C. Fetal malpresentation
    D. Suspected fetal distress
    E. Third trimester bleeding

72. Immediate care of the newborn infant would include all of the following EXCEPT:
    A. Suction mouth
    B. Provide warmth
    C. Assess heart rate
    D. Tactile stimulation
    E. Position head upward

73. A small for gestational age fetus which is asymmetrically grown should arouse suspicion of:
    A. Small parents
    B. Maternal diabetes
    C. Chronic hypertension
    D. Chromosomal disorder
    E. late onset placental dysfunction

74. Which laboratory test on newborn blood is not routine?
    A. VDRL
    B. T4/TSH
    C. Glucose
    D. Calcium
    E. Hematocrit

75. A medication given to the newborn to promote healing of the umbilical cord would be:
    A. Dextrose
    B. Naloxone
    C. Triple dye
    D. Vitamin K
    E. Tetracycline

76. An expected change in the maternal blood count during the first three postpartum days would be:
    A. Leukocytosis
    B. Eosinophilia
    C. Lymphocytopenia
    D. Thrombocytopenia
    E. Increased hematocrit

77. Routine postpartum care should include searching for all of the following EXCEPT:
    A. Fever
    B. Anemia
    C. Diabetes
    D. Depression
    E. Thrombophlebitis

78. Which statement is true about insulin therapy during pregnancy?
    A. The drug crosses the placenta easily.
    B. A single daily dose is often adequate.
    C. Doses are decreased as gestation advances.
    D. A recombinant DNA preparation is preferred.
    E. Insulin should be avoided during the first trimester.

79. Appropriate studies to be performed on a gestational-onset diabetic would be:
    A. Fetal ultrasonography
    B. Fetal echocardiography
    C. Maternal creatinine clearance
    D. Amniotic fluid alphafetoprotein
    E. Maternal glycosylated hemoglobin A,C

80. A twin fetus is at increased risk for each of the following complications EXCEPT:
    A. Stillbirth
    B. Anomalies
    C. Macrosomia
    D. Malpresentation
    E. Umbilical cord entanglement

81. Searching at delivery for a cause of stillbirth should include all the following EXCEPT:
    A. Cervical culture
    B. External fetal anomalies
    C. Umbilical vessel inspection
    D. Fetal cells for karyotyping
    E. Obtain a consent for autopsy

82. The most common cause of premature labor is:
    A. Unknown
    B. Dehydration
    C. Polyhydramnios
    D. Incompetent cervix
    E. Ruptured membranes

83. Which form of therapy is often most effective for patients with premature labor?
    A. Bedrest
    B. Cervical cerclage
    C. Intravenous ampicillin
    D. Oral beta adrenergic agents
    E. Intramuscular corticosteroid

84. Initial evaluation of the patient with third trimester bleeding should NOT include a:
    A. Pap smear
    B. Platelet count
    C. fetal heart rate tracing
    D. Serum fibrinogen level
    E. Ultrasound examination

85. Management of hemorrhage shock should include:
    A. Infusing nitroglycerin
    B. Placing a central venous line
    C. Elevating the head of the bed
    D. Transfusing with whole blood
    E. Expanding the plasma with Lactated ringer's

86. An infant born to a postterm rather than term pregnancy is more likely to have:
    A. Meconium aspiration
    B. Cardiac malformations
    C. Symmetric growth retardation
    D. Umbilical cord entanglements
    E. Group B streptococcal infection

87. Evaluation of a fetus during active labor having variable decelerations should include all of the following EXCEPT:
    A. Amnioinfusion
    B. External version
    C. Fetal scalp stimulation
    D. Fetal acoustic stimulation
    E. Determination of fetal presentation

88. A fetal heart rate pattern most suggestive of long term central nervous system dysfunction would be:
    A. Late decelerations
    B. Severe bradycardia
    C. Persistent tachycardia
    D. Repetitive variable decelerations
    E. Unexplained loss of beat-to-beat variability

89. The most probable cause of excessive hemorrhage shortly after a vaginal delivery would be:
    A. Uterine atony
    B. A coagulopathy
    C. Tear of the cervix
    D. Concealed pelvic hematoma
    E. Retained placental fragments

90. The most likely cause of maternal fever on the first morning after cesarean section would be:
    A. Atelectasis
    B. Endomyometritis
    C. Noninfectious mastitis
    D. Urinary tract infection
    E. Septic thrombophlebitis

91. Conditions to consider before performing a postpartum sterilization include all of the following EXCEPT:
    A. A signed permit
    B. Normal coagulogram
    C. Negative pap smear
    D. The infants' well being
    E. The patient awareness of hormonal suppression therapy

92. A patient known to be 9 weeks pregnant is found to be spotting, with a closed cervix and uterine size equal to menstrual dates. The primary diagnosis would be:
    A. Missed abortion
    B. Ectopic pregnancy
    C. Complete abortion
    D. Threatened abortion
    E. Incomplete abortion

93. The most appropriate form of therapy would be:
    A. Oral methotrexate
    B. Expectant management
    C. Dilation and curettage
    D. Dilation and evacuation
    E. Laparoscopic salpingostomy

94. A patient with acute pelvic pain has a low grade fever, Nontender uterus and negative beta hCG test, and negative urinalysis. The most probable diagnosis would be:
    A. Salpingitis
    B. Appendicitis
    C. Missed abortion
    D. Ectopic pregnancy
    E. Ruptured ovarian cyst

95. The risk of recurrence for many major anomalies is:
    A. 0.2 - 0.4%
    B. 2-4%
    C. 12-14%
    D. 20-25%
    E. 50%

96. An abnormally low maternal serum alphafetoprotein (MSAFP) result is associated with:
    A. Twins
    B. Stillbirth
    C. Trisomy 21
    D. Abdominal wall defect
    E. Open neural tube defect

97.   Which statement is true about drug effects on the fetus?
      A.   Facial clefts should be excluded
      B.   Many are associated with specific anomalies
      C.   The risk of major anomalies is 2-4%, regardless of any drugs
      D.   An amniocentesis for karyotyping is helpful.
      E.   Teratogenic risk is synonymous with minor and major birth defects

98.   Limitations with antepartum fetal testing include all of the following EXCEPT:
      A.   Falsely abnormal results are high
      B.   Results are not immediately available
      C.   Results are often unable to predict a placental abruption
      D.   Results are often unable to predict an umbilical cord entanglement
      E.   Underlying fetal conditions may change and lead to different results

99.   An indication for an advanced or targeted ultrasound scan would be to:
      A.   Rule out twins
      B.   Localize the placenta
      C.   Evaluate polyhydramnios
      D.   Confirm a breech presentation
      E.   Guide the needle during amniocentesis

100. Signs of fetal maturity would include all of the following EXCEPT:
      A.   Amniotic fluid phosphatidylglycerol
      B.   Amniotic fluid luetin/sphingomyelin
      C.   Estimated fetal weight greater than six pounds
      D.   Gestational age $\geq$ 39 weeks and grade III placenta
      E.   Gestational age $\geq$ 39 weeks and biparietal diameter > 12 mm

101. Chronic hypertension may be defined as:
      A.   A blood pressure $\geq$ 160/110 mmHg
      B.   Hypertension before 20 weeks gestation
      C.   Hypertension accompanied with 5g protein/24 h
      D.   Hypertension being present during the present and past pregnancies
      E.   Blood pressure elevations on at least two occasions during the pregnancy

102. Laboratory studies used to evaluate the patient with presumed pre-eclampsia include:
      A.   Hematocrit
      B.   Platelet count
      C.   Prothrombin time
      D.   Serum hemoglobin A_1C
      E.   Serum transaminase levels

103. Which of the following intrapartum fetal heart rate patterns is reassuring?
   A. Tachycardia
   B. Accelerations
   C. Late decelerations
   D. Variable decelerations
   E. Decreased beat-to-beat variability

104. Management of an abnormal intrapartum fetal heart rate pattern would include all of the following EXCEPT:
   A. Administer naloxone
   B. Administer oxygen
   C. Discontinue oxytocin
   D. Change maternal position
   E. Examine for imminent delivery

ANSWERS TO QUESTIONS

1. C	33. C	65. E	97. C
2. C	34. C	66. D	98. B
3. C	35. E	67. B	99. C
4. E	36. B	68. C	100. C
5. A	37. A	69. B	101. B
6. B	38. B	70. B	102. D
7. E	39. B	71. A	103. B
8. C	40. B	72. E	104. A
9. D	41. D	73. E	
10. C	42. C	74. D	
11. B	43. C	75. C	
12. A	44. B	76. E	
13. B	45. A	77. C	
14. E	46. D	78. D	
15. D	47. C	79. D	
16. B	48. D	80. C	
17. C	49. E	81. A	
18. C	50. A	82. A	
19. A	51. B	83. A	
20. D	52. C	84. A	
21. B	53. C	85. E	
22. E	54. D	86. A	
23. A	55. D	87. B	
24. B	56. A	88. E	
25. A	57. D	89. A	
26. C	58. C	90. B	
27. E	59. E	91. E	
28. E	60. A	92. D	
29. D	61. D	93. B	
30. A	62. A, B, D	94. A	
31. G	63. A	95. B	
32. F	64. D	96. C	